Four Strong Winds

UNDERSTANDING THE GROWING CHALLENGES TO HEALTH CARE

Michael B. Decter •

Published in 2000 by Stoddart Publishing Co. Limited
34 Lesmill Road, Toronto, Canada M3B 2T6
180 Varick Street, 9th Floor, New York, New York 10014

Distributed in Canada by:
General Distribution Services Ltd.
325 Humber College Blvd., Toronto, Canada M9W 7C3
Tel. (416) 213-1919   Fax (416) 213-1917
Email cservice@genpub.com

Distributed in the U.S. by:
General Distribution Services Inc.
PMB 128, 4500 Witmer Industrial Estates, Niagara Falls, New York 14305-1386
Toll-free Tel.1-800-805-1083   Toll-free Fax 1-800-481-6207
Email gdsinc@genpub.com

04   03   02   01   00   1   2   3   4   5

Canadian Cataloguing in Publication Data
Decter, Michael B.
Four strong winds: understanding the growing challenges to health care
Includes bibliographical references and index.

ISBN 0-7737-3224-1

1. Medical care — Canada. 2. Medical policy — Canada. I. Title.
RA395.C3D38 2000   362.1'0971   C00-930035-X

U.S. Cataloguing in Publication Data
(Library of Congress Standards)
Decter, Michael B.
Four strong winds: understanding the growing challenges to
health care / Michael B. Decter. — 1st ed.
[256]p.: cm.
Includes bibliographic references and index.
Summary: Examines questions such as public vs. private health care,
the future of hospitals, the impact of new technologies,
and costs and needs of an aging population.

ISBN 0-7737-3224-1

1. Medical policy. 2. World Health. 3. Medical economics.
4. Health Surveys. I. Title.
362.1   21   2000   CIP

Jacket design: Bill Douglas @ The Bang
Text design: Tannice Goddard

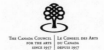

THE CANADA COUNCIL | LE CONSEIL DES ARTS
FOR THE ARTS | DU CANADA
SINCE 1957 | DEPUIS 1957

*We acknowledge for their financial support of our
publishing program the Canada Council, the Ontario Arts
Council, and the Government of Canada through the
Book Publishing Industry Development Program (BPIDP).*

Printed and bound in Canada

To the tens of millions of men and women throughout the world who have devoted their lives to caring for their fellow human beings. As health-care services change and transform, I hope you retain your humanity and compassion.

Contents

Foreword

This book has a direct and simple origin. As I have travelled to many cities and countries to learn, speak, and consult, I am asked two questions on every single occasion:

◇ What are the forces driving change in health-care systems?
◇ Where are these forces taking our health systems?

This book is my answer.

Acknowledgements

For the past six years, since the publication of my first book, *Healing Medicare: Managing Health System Change the Canadian Way*, I have travelled rather relentlessly as a health consultant and speaker on matters of health reform. For three years these travels were as managing director, Canada, for APM Inc. More recently, I have toiled as managing director of my own consultancy, Michael Decter and Associates Ltd. Since December of 1997, I have also served as the volunteer chair of the board of the Canadian Institute for Health Information. I have often been invited to speak on matters of health-system management and health policy.

Through my travels and encounters with health-policy thinkers and managers from all over the globe, my own views have expanded, changed, and sharpened. During my journeys, I have become intrigued by the forces driving change in health care and by the direction those forces are taking us. There is a curiosity among the makers of health policy, health-care providers, managers, and concerned citizens about the future prospects for health services. There is also a great deal of fear. The recent hectic pace of change has been jarring for many.

My purpose in this book is to articulate the forces as I see them and examine their impact. As you will rapidly discover, it is not a scholarly book (some day I will write one). It is intended to help those whose lives are touched by health-care systems to better manage and survive change by better understanding forces underlying it. It is also my hope that I can encourage health-policy makers and managers to look to the experiences of other sectors, particularly other service industries, for ideas that can be adapted to the realm of health. If those in the health-care service trenches can glimpse the future, it can only aid their cause.

Amid the ceaseless pressures of my consulting work, this book has been written in fits and starts. It took shape in hotels late at night, on bumpy airplane flights, and, surreptitiously, I hope, in boring meetings. It is the product of late evenings, early mornings, and weekends. It is truly a "stolen moments" book. I hope the staccato style resulting from its genesis does not distract too much from its broader purpose.

As I did with my previous book, I owe a significant debt to Dr. Robert Maxwell and the King Edward's Hospital Fund for London. Dr. Maxwell ably led the King's Fund as its chief executive for seventeen inspiring years before retiring in 1997. The King's Fund International Seminar has been a powerful stimulus to continue my study of how health-care systems are evolving.

As well, the Four Country Conferences in which I have participated (the four countries are Germany, the Netherlands, Canada, and the United States) provided me with insight into North American and European reforms. Dr. Kieke Okma remains the founder and driving force of these conferences, which I attended in 1995 (The Netherlands), 1996 (Canada), 1997 (Germany), and 1998 (United States), gaining access to leading health thinkers and opportunities to test my ideas. Sadly, I missed the 1999 conference in Sydney because of a family illness. I am grateful to my colleagues who have helped share my thinking through these conferences. In particular, Professor James Morone of Brown University provided a constructive reaction to some of these ideas at Yale University in the summer of 1998. His critique of "Decter's doppel-ganger" (my evil twin) was insightful and thought provoking.

My former colleagues at APM are a remarkably energetic, intelligent, and driven group. The support of Arthur Spiegel provided important encouragement in his best "take it to the next level" and "just do it" style. As well, my large debt to a wide array of APM people for their insights is gratefully acknowledged. In particular, my former Toronto colleagues Myrna Francis, Will Falk, and Jan Norris provided a sounding board for many of these ideas.

A special thanks to Professor Linda Aiken, director of the Center for Health Services and Policy Research at the University of Pennsylvania; Claire Fagin, former dean of Nursing and former president of the University of Pennsylvania and the Rockefeller Foundation. Through their efforts I spent an informative, reflective, and productive four days at the marvellous Rockefeller Study and Conference Center in Bellagio, Italy, in 1996. The conference "Planning an Integrational Study of the Outcomes of Hospital Restructuring" provided stimulation and lively debate. The new friends I made in Bellagio have expanded my depth of knowledge and understanding, particularly in the field of nursing.

My friends and colleagues, Dr. Judith Shamian of Mount Sinai Hospital in Toronto and Dr. Kieke Okma of the Dutch Ministry of Health, were both of great help and support in completion of this book. More important, they have both challenged my thinking and made me dig deeper and consider the evidence more seriously. For their diligence and assistance I am most grateful.

A special thank you to Annie Balant and Sharon Laughlin. Without them these words would not be on these pages.

My children, Geneviève and Riel, remain my inspiration. They ask the rude questions and treat my answers with the certain skepticism of their youth. Watching their comfort with the new technologies of the Internet and the new performance standards of our service economy has taught me a great deal. They have my love, my respect, and my gratitude.

Introduction

For most of the twentieth century, health care has been the world's largest local, or "cottage," industry. Communities all over the world have built hospitals. Societies have trained doctors and nurses, and funded health-care services — services that are highly prized by citizens. We seek relief from our pains and we search out cures for our illnesses.

It is not surprising, therefore, that health care is a priority for public and private spending in all nations. Governments, communities, and employers have organized systems to finance health-care services. But it has been only in the last decade or so that serious efforts to organize integrated systems of care delivery have gained momentum. This shift from systems of finance to systems of delivery is profound. It is an unprecedented change, both in its direction and in its speed.

The long-established medical guild is under siege as doctors are questioned about everything they have long regarded as sacred. So too, the are nurses, who feel set upon as their profession is restructured, hospital by hospital, nation by nation. The old ways of both physician and nursing care are being altered forever.

Health-care delivery is undergoing rapid changes, evolutionary and revolutionary. Much has been written about the nature of these changes, country by country. Among the emergent new approaches are the integrated delivery systems in the United States, Crown health enterprises in New Zealand, and purchasing authorities in the United Kingdom. However, very little has been written about the actual experience of these new organizations. Is the integration of health services working? What are its early consequences — for patients? For providers? For communities?

Even less has been written about the powerful societal forces driving these changes. Studying health-system change without understanding these forces misses the dynamic motion that underlies the upheaval. It is like trying to teach sailing without discussing winds. As a young student, I taught sailing during my summers, to small children and sometimes to their parents. The first essential lessons in sailing are not about the boat but about the winds. No sailor can function without understanding the many clues to the directions of winds: the wind on the water, the wind in the rigging, the patterns of clouds, the shape of the land. . . . Knowing the true wind, with its shifting, changing force and direction, is a challenge with which all sailors must contend. Without knowledge of the winds, one is merely an "accidental" sailor — and will never really be in control of the boat.

Of course, understanding the boat is essential as well. To leave the metaphor and come back to health care, this means understanding the vessels that provide it — institutions and organizations that have often been built over long periods of time and are deeply rooted in the values of the communities they serve.

Those responsible for managing the great changes in health care face a highly complicated, challenging task. Health-care systems are some of the most complex organizations we have devised as a species. They are buffeted by strong winds of change. Like sailors, their managers must understand the winds blowing against their rigging if they are to contend with them successfully. Without this understanding, they are no better off than the accidental sailor.

There is no shortage of accidental health reformers. U.S. President Bill Clinton might be the most prominent; his proposed reforms were not rooted in an understanding of the forces driving change — nor did they reflect American values well. The reforms inevitably failed.

Clinton fundamentally misunderstood the power of the coalitions that support the current U.S. health-care system. Although health-insurance coverage for all Americans had political appeal, opponents of the model proposed by Clinton were easily able to portray it as overly bureaucratic and governmental. No matter how unfair this character-ization might have been, it stuck. A consumerist public with rising expectations of quality and speed in health services did not believe these demands would be met by the Clinton approach, quality and speed not being virtues most Americans associate with their government.

Much of the one-time efficiency the Clinton reforms sought has now been achieved by health maintenance organizations. The goal of univer-sal coverage has drifted further from the achievable as more Americans than ever — some 40 million — lack any health coverage at all, and tens of millions more have inadequate insurance. This situation persists after the longest period of economic prosperity in American history.

Across the industrialized world, health systems — which consisted largely of hospitals and doctors — were fuelled by more and more fund-ing in the four decades following World War II. Through the 1950s to the mid-1980s, billions and billions of dollars poured in. Growth in health spending averaged well above 10% — higher than inflation, higher than population growth. The late 1980s and 1990s marked a sudden change in the approach to health financing in industrialized countries. Hospital funding has been frozen or reduced. Now, health managers and planners must reshape health-care delivery organizations to be lighter, more dollar efficient, and yet of higher quality and more responsive to consumers.

Like early naval architects working to design ships that could sail closer and closer to the wind, health leaders must design health services to be delivered closer and closer to the populations they serve. Like the square-rigged galleons of centuries past, the stand-alone general hospital is increasingly an anachronism.

The winds of change do not blow steadily, but shift as they bump up against existing health systems. They blow in more than one direction at a time — at times they are in conflict, and at other times they reinforce each other. Sometimes they are gentle breezes, and sometimes they are howling hurricanes. At times, existing health-delivery systems must claw their way to windward, fighting for each inch of room to deliver services. At other times, the winds are behind them; these favourable winds will waft lighter, leaner delivery systems swiftly into the future.

Not all change is for the better. There are always casualties in a period of reform. In all countries, the disruptions of reform are creating problems for patients and providers. It is a turbulent era in health care as the winds of change blow both good and ill into our health-care systems even as they profoundly alter how we think about health and how we deliver health care.

These winds are global. They do not abate at national borders. They do not respect tradition or the centuries-old values of physicians and nurses. They do not bend to the will of politicians.

What are these powerful forces? What are the north, south, east, and west winds blowing through global health systems, compelling their rapid transformation? I have identified four important forces of change, as follows:

◇ powerful new ideas, including a paradigm shift in health policy from providing individual health care services to managing costs to endeavouring to manage the health status of populations;
◇ a consumer revolution — what the public wants is quality, speed, affordability, and appropriateness, as well as accessibility; what it needs is shaped by demographics;
◇ the technological transformation of health-services delivery, driven

by silicon-chip-enhanced information management, new drugs, the biotechnological revolution, and changing clinical practice; and

◇ financial pressure from employers and from governments to deliver more services, more efficiently — driven by global competitive pressures.

Let us consider each of these forces briefly.

Powerful New Ideas

There are both radical new ideas and radical old ideas at large in the world of health today. The idea that health intervention should be as much or more about enhancing health status than curing disease is not new, but it is a paradigm that has gained tremendous force in the major industrialized countries in the past two decades. In 1974, Marc Lalonde, then Canadian Health Minister, issued a key report that made an effective case for broader determinants of health. Over the next two decades, other industrialized nations followed the Canadian lead. Each in its own fashion has embraced this approach; its implementation, however, both in Canada and elsewhere, has been less rapid. The old ways of health show resistance to even the strongest forces.

Vast investments in new drugs and technologies have yielded great advances — yet diminishing returns. The potential of this realm remains great, yet unlocking it has proven elusive. As diseases such as cancer remain stubbornly resistant to cure, our attention has turned sharply to prevention. With regard to cancer, for example, the linking of many causal factors, particularly smoking and diet, to various forms of cancer has given health advocates the momentum needed to move the system toward this new paradigm. Health promotion has gained millions of allies.

The idea of measuring health by the life expectancy of a population, and particularly its disability-free years of life, has also gained great momentum in the world health community. No one is suggesting that we abandon accounting for how we treat illness and cure disease.

However, we are witnessing a much greater focus on the health of a population, the epidemiology of disease, and the search for root causes that can be altered. Chief among these are income level (health rises with wealth), lifestyle choices, and the safety of the general environment. The World Bank report of 1993 marked a watershed in the movement toward investing in improving health rather than in simply treating illness.

In the United States, the health-care debate of the 1990s was dominated by the concept of managed care — and the reality of its implementation. Health maintenance organizations have been the controversial vehicles for this massive experiment. Has managed care stalled at managed cost? Did it achieve a one-time saving by removing excess capacity only to fall victim to its own success?

There are other powerful ideas shaping health policy, particularly the notion of competition as a means of improving efficiency, and the idea of more integrated approaches to care delivery. Each of these ideas will be explored in greater deal in Chapter 1.

Changing Public Expectations

Changing public expectations are the second powerful driver of reform. The era of provider domination in health has endured for several centuries. But this tradition, which was based largely on information monopolies, is giving way to the age of the empowered consumer. Consumers can reach out through the Internet to drkoop.com, fire up a CD-ROM, read one of hundreds of new books, or simply turn on the television to obtain information on a scale unimaginable less than a decade ago. We can now know what it is that our bodies are confronting. We can know our risk factors.

Public expectations combine with changing demographics as a force for change. Our health needs change as we age — and we are aging, all of us, one year at a time. This the best educated generation, ever.

We are confronted in every other walk of life by a rapid increase in the pace of activity. We no longer have the patience to line up in our bank branches — automated teller machines have proliferated. At gas stations, we have self-service pumps. Automated-checkout machinery has sped up the supermarket experience. Fifty channels on television — soon to be five hundred. Five million Web sites on the Internet — soon to be fifty million. In every walk of life the consumer's desire for speed has brought about a transformation, be it fast food or fast entertainment.

There is also greater demand for quality. The revolution that swept through the car industry several decades ago has, in the last several years, come to health-care delivery. Chapter 2 explores the wants and needs of today's new consumer as they relate to health care, specifically the changing public expectations regarding quality, speed, and appropriateness.

New, Chip-Driven Technology

Perhaps the most profound of the societal forces driving change in the delivery of health care worldwide is technological change — specifically, the coming of the digital age. The ubiquitous silicon chip, which has transformed our ability to obtain, store, and manage information, is affecting health care in a myriad of ways. Other technological advances have had an important effect, too — for example, our vastly enhanced ability to scan and image the human body in much less intrusive ways and with much less risk to patients than ever before. And new wonder drugs, although at a greater cost for each than previously. But it is the silicon chip, and its unprecedented effect on our ability to manage information, that is at the centre of the technology revolution in health care. Chapter 3 reviews this interplay of technology and change.

Financial Pressures

Finally, there is the fiscal crisis — the big squeeze. As government debt and deficits reached unsustainable levels across the industrialized countries in the late 1980s and early 1990s, health-care cost containment became a central issue — one that became even more pressing in several nations as fiscal situations tightened with recessions.

The form that cost containment has taken differs according to the nation and its particular system. In most countries, where financial responsibility for health-care services rests with the state, the government has brought about change and rationalization in how these services are delivered and managed. In the United States, where responsibility for health insurance rests primarily with private employers, this rationalization has been largely a marketplace phenomenon. Chapter 4 reviews the relationship between money and its restriction, affected health care, and discusses the recent move toward reinvestment of funds as we enter the twenty-first century.

These are the four powerful winds blowing through global health care: new ideas and a different vision of health; a more demanding and knowledgeable public; advances in technology — in particular chip-based technology; and a desire for greater affordability and value for money. These forces are bringing about phenomenal and rapid change in health-care delivery as we know it. They offer the potential for great constructive change, as well as the certainty of a significant disruption of the existing order.

The Structure of This Book

Part I explores each of the forces in great detail — giving the "navigators" of health care a chance to understand the contours and the velocity of each wind.

Part II examines the impact of these winds on some of the most important and familiar aspects of existing health systems: hospitals, physician care, nursing care, and drugs. The emergence of new organizations and approaches — such as managed-care organizations and disease-state management — is also probed. The final two chapters in this part examine the implications of the forces of change on public health and care in the home.

In Part III, we travel through five countries to explore emerging realities. Several case studies are examined as examples of leading integrated-health systems. What is the real-life experience of the people living through these changes in various places? What lessons can the rest of the world learn from the early results of each nation's efforts to change?

Part IV probes some of the more complex concepts of the health-care revolution — concepts that I believe will profoundly affect the shape of the sector in the next century — in more detail. First up is the emergence of the health-care consumer; the consumer revolution in health is a real key to the future path of this sector. Next is the little-discussed concept of organized effort to manage *demand* for health care. In health services, the intersection of supply and demand is hotly contested ground. The battle between forces trying to manage demand and the rise of the consumer will shape health services in this new century.

Next is an exploration of the emerging world of silicon-chip-driven health companies, and how these new ventures are reshaping health services. There follow discussions of the evidence revolution, disease-state management, and the world of human genetic research — once the realm of science fiction and increasingly a routine aspect of science and medicine.

Will these winds become a hurricane of destruction, or steady, dependable westerlies pushing health-care systems smoothly in sensible directions? Only time and the vantage point of a future time will fully answer that question. But the greater one's understanding of the winds driving this change, the more skilful and successful one will be as a sailor. In health care, policy makers, managers, providers, and consumers can all benefit from greater insight into the winds of change. With an understanding of these forces, change can be managed more effectively and its impacts survived. With insight, the benefits of change can be harnessed to the challenge of health for all and effective health care for those who need it.

PART I •

The Four Strong Winds of Change

1

•

Powerful New Ideas

No army can withstand the strength of an idea whose time has come.

— VICTOR HUGO

In the post–World War II era, the industrialized nations were gripped with a fervour for growth. Economic growth was welcomed as a way to put distance between the deprivation of war and the new era of prosperity. In every area of society, newer and bigger were also seen as better. More became more virtuous.

Health care was no exception. There was a building boom in hospitals and medical schools. The quest for new treatments, better drugs, and better medical devices was unending. The appetite of health-care providers for more and more money seemed insatiable — yet the economy of the 1950s and 1960s was able to support growth on this scale.

The defining market for most health-care product development in the Western world was the United States, which had in place such a fragmented system of health-care delivery that there was no real possibility of containing costs. Between 1975 and 1999, health-care spending in the United States rose from a few hundred billion to more than a trillion dollars. The percentage of the gross national product (GNP) devoted to health rose from 8.4% to 14.3% over the same period. In 1975, one dollar of every twelve in the American economy was spent on health care; by 1999, this amount had climbed to one dollar of every seven.

This rapid increase in health-care spending was not solely an American phenomenon, although the United States led the world in both percentage of GNP and in absolute dollars spent on health services. In virtually every industrialized country, health costs climbed faster than either inflation or economic growth — or even than the two combined.

As costs skyrocketed, the concept that "more and bigger equals better" came under sustained scrutiny and mounting criticism. New ideas began to be discussed by health policy thinkers. As new answers were sought by corporate and government leaders, the appetite for new thinking expanded. The debate broadened to include not just health experts but also the larger community of those who provide health services and those who pay for them. Questions hotly debated included not only the cost of care but also its value — concepts that differ in important ways — and also how it is organized and delivered.

Out of this climate of debate and dissatisfaction with the status quo were born a host of new ideas and new ways of looking at health care — and even at the concept of health itself. These ideas form the first of the four "winds of change" that are redefining the world of health care today. Taken together, they are a powerful force; health policy makers throughout the developed world have embraced them — for better or for worse.

Broader Determinants of Health

The first of these new ideas to take root was a broader perspective on what exactly constitutes health. The focus moved from health *services* to health *status*. By the mid-1970s, a quiet revolution was under way in many parts of the world. A new view was taking hold, one that incorporated the concept of diminishing returns on investments in health-care treatment. The realization was dawning that most of the gains in the postwar era came not from enhanced spending on the *treatment* of disease but from a set of broader determinants of health, most of which related to the *prevention* of disease, such as public policy, income, and lifestyle choices.

In Canada, this new view was articulated in a 1974 report by the Health Minister, Marc Lalonde. The Lalonde Report argued for a "health-field concept," which it described in terms of four broad elements: human biology, environment, lifestyle, and health-care organization. The report argued that the last of these elements, more commonly known as the health-care system, accounted for most of Canada's spending in health, but ultimately shouldered less of the burden of preventing illness than the other three determinants.

The report defined these four determinants as follows:

Human Biology
The Human Biology element includes all those aspects of health, both physical and mental, which are developed within the human body as a consequence of the basic biology of man and the organic make-up of the individual. This element includes the genetic inheritance of the individual, the processes of maturation and aging, and the many complex internal systems in the body. . . . [T]he health implications of human biology are numerous, varied and serious, and the things that can go wrong . . . are legion. This element contributes to all kinds of ill health and mortality, including many chronic diseases (such as arthritis, diabetes, atherosclerosis, cancer)

and others (genetic disorders, congenital malformation, mental retardation).

Environment
The Environment category includes all those matters related to health which are external to the human body and over which the individual has little or no control. Individuals cannot, by themselves, ensure that goods, drugs, cosmetics, devices, water supply, etc., are safe and uncontaminated; that the health hazards of air, water and noise pollution are controlled; that the spread of communicable diseases is prevented; that effective garbage and sewage disposal is carried out; and that the social environment, including the rapid changes in it, do not have harmful effects on health.

Lifestyle
The Lifestyle category . . . consists of the aggregation of decisions by individuals which affect their health and over which they more or less have control. . . . Personal decisions and habits that are bad, from a health point of view, create self-imposed risks. When those risks result in illness or death, the victim's lifestyle can be said to have contributed to, or caused, his own illness or death.

Health-Care Organization
The fourth category consists of the quantity, quality, arrangement, nature, and relationships of people and resources in the provision of health care. It includes medical practice, nursing, hospitals, nursing homes, medical drugs, public and community health-care services, ambulances, dental treatment, and other health services such as optometry, chiropractics, and podiatry. This fourth element is what is generally defined as the health-care system.

The Lalonde Report outlined how the concept of a four-part health field can be used to analyze social policy:

. . . the Concept permits a system of analysis by which any question can be examined under the four elements in order to assess their relative significance and interaction. For example, the underlying causes of death from traffic accidents can be found to be due mainly to risks taken by individuals, with lesser importance given to the design of cars and roads, and to the availability of emergency treatment; human biology has little or no significance in this area. In order of importance, therefore, lifestyle, environment and health care organization contribute to traffic deaths in the proportions of something like 75%, 20%, and 5% respectively. This analysis permits program planners to focus their attention on the most important contributing factors. Similar assessments of the relative importance of contributing factors can be made for many other health problems.

Over the past twenty years each of the industrial nations has tackled this issue in its own way. The United Kingdom adopted "health gain" as its slogan. The United States adopted specific health goals and formulated policy in the language of population health. In virtually every major developed nation, the shift from equating health with health services to taking a broader view has been legitimized by a major national commission, study, or forum. In countries such as Australia, Canada, and the United States, in which two levels of government have some stake in health-care policy, such national study efforts have often been replicated at the provincial or state level. In Canada, a dozen royal commissions, councils, and studies reproduced the Lalonde thinking over a fifteen-year span. In British Columbia, a royal commission produced similar results, and in Ontario, the Premier's Council on Health Strategy did the same.

The theme of all of these reports has altered little since 1974. They all stress the importance of broader determinants of health, often categorizing them in much the same way that did Lalonde.

Twenty-five years after the Lalonde Report, a group of researchers led by Sholom Glouberman researched the impacts in Canada of the Lalonde thinking. The researchers produced a "report card" that ranked Canada's progress in each of the four fields. Their conclusion was that Canada had performed better, in terms of promoting overall health, in the lifestyle field than in any of the others.

The Lalonde Report Card

Environment Tool: legislation B–	**Lifestyle** Tool: social marketing A–
Human Biology Tool: research B	**Health-Care Organization** Tool: reorganization C+

Source: Health and Welfare Canada, *A New Perspective on the Health of Canadians: A Working Document*, 1974.

In the face of this new perspective, many health reformers and policy makers worldwide adopted the view that a better balance between treatment and health promotion/prevention was needed. The concept of broader determinants of health, once embraced, meant a serious shift in spending patterns and priorities.

Some of the practical implications of rebalancing the system this way are obvious: increased emphasis on immunization, focus on reducing tobacco use, improvements in transportation safety such as seat belts and motorcycle helmets, etc. But the full implications of this revolution in thinking are much broader, encompassing various kinds of advocacy for a more balanced approach to health and health care.

More and more, we are moving beyond a definition of health as merely the absence of ill health. The World Health Organization (WHO) calls it "a complete state of physical, mental, social, and emotional well-being." Health is a resource for living that enables people of all ages to realize their hopes and needs, and to change or cope with the environments around them.

Competition

The idea of competition as a drive to efficiency is another new notion in health care — new, that is, everywhere but in the United States, where it has been a cornerstone of health-care policy for some time. Until recently it has been wholly rejected in other nations, where market and competition were seen as the trappings of an ability-to-pay system embraced only by Americans. No other nations were keen to develop the large uninsured population that was seen as a consequence of such a system. The principle of solidarity — that benefits should not be linked to ability to pay — led health-care policy thinkers and managers in countries such as the United Kingdom and Canada away from markets in their search for policies. All industrialized nations took universal insurance coverage as a basic starting point — except the United States, where it has proven an impossible political challenge.

However, the notion of *internal* markets, or public competition — that is, the use of market mechanisms to allocate resources without moving away from a fundamentally public system — gained enormous momentum in several countries in the 1980s and 1990s. British Prime Minister Margaret Thatcher introduced the notion of the purchaser/provider split to shake up the by-then constipated British National Health Service. In Scandinavia, internal markets have been seen as a means of adjusting more rapidly to consumer needs. In New Zealand, radical ideas based on internal market reforms took hold rapidly, but have subsequently been modified and even reversed.

This notion of internal markets for public competition — the so-called purchaser/provider split — gained prominence because political leaders were fed up with slow-moving, expensive health bureaucracies. Their high cost and resistance to change led ministers of health to consider radical measures. Creating competition among health-care providers was seen as a way of making the system more responsive. In the United Kingdom, this movement toward competition has involved turning some responsibility for purchasing specialized health services over to general practitioners. In other countries, particularly in

Scandinavia, dollars now follow patients as they move among local or county health systems. The principle behind both of these kinds of reform is to bring the competitive drive of a marketplace to bear on the provision of health services without abandoning a single-payer public system as the primary mode of health-care delivery. In both examples, the "solidarity" principle is respected — health-care costs are borne by the society, not by the individual. How this situation was achieved in various nations provides an interesting overview of possible models.

In the United Kingdom, the separation of provision of care from payment for care operates in two ways. First, the National Health Service directs funds to health-services purchasing authorities, who enter into contracts with newly independent trust hospitals and physician groups. The hospitals contract to provide services of a certain quality and price, and purchasing authorities are able to direct business to the most effi-cient, highest-quality institutions. Second, under the system known as GP fundholding, groups of six or more general practitioners control budgets to purchase specialty services on behalf of their patients.

One interesting indicator of how these changes have shaken up the traditional U.K. system, in which specialists had long been the most powerful group, is illustrated by the observation, passed on to me by a British health manager, that before the introduction of GP fundholding, Christmas cards were traditionally sent by general practitioners to specialists. Since the introduction of GP fundholding, it has been the specialists who send Christmas cards to the general practitioners. Clearly, a genuine power shift has occurred, and with it an enormous increase in the responsiveness of the system. A general practitioner with a fixed budget to buy, for example, hip replacements is likely to shop locally rather than sending his patients, as had been the traditional referral pattern, to a farther-off academic medical centre, which might easily have prices 20% to 30% higher.

New Zealand adopted, for a time, an extreme variation on the public competition model. The approach, which has since been abandoned, separated the purchasing of care from its provision completely. Four health purchasing authorities and twenty-three Crown health enterprises (CHEs), which delivered health-care services on a corporate model, were created. Their shares were jointly held by the Treasury Department and by the Department of Crown Enterprises. Funding flowed from the Department of Health to the four purchasing authorities, which in turn bought services from the CHEs on the open market. The CHEs delivered health services to the New Zealand public.

No full formal evaluation of the New Zealand public-competition or internal-market model was ever undertaken. There was some suggestion that many of the Crown-held enterprises never became self-sufficient or able to cope with the diminished health budget. A strong case was made for consolidating the system into fewer than twenty-three CHEs. But before any tinkering with the system could occur, a major overhaul was brought about by a change of government. The public-competition model, while never fully evaluated from an organizational perspective, failed in the all-important court of public opinion. It has been displaced by a return to less extreme models of health-care service organization. (For a more detailed case study from New Zealand, see Chapter 13.)

Population density plays a major role in the success of a public-competition model of health care. In urban areas, or in countries such as the United Kingdom where population densities are high, it is possible for both individuals and purchasers to choose alternative providers. Where populations are more spread out, as in Canada, the tendency instead has been toward more comprehensive health organizations.

At the core of this idea of competition is the notion that the purchasing and the provision of care should be separate. An independent health-services purchaser creates a market, so as a system moves toward a competition-based model, it moves away from the concept of insured services and toward the concept of purchased services. No longer is the physician dominant in determining medical necessity, but rather a group of purchasers and providers interact in constructing a package of health-related services to be purchased at a particular price. Competition among providers leads to more efficiency in this model.

The purchasing approach has been criticized for transforming health services into a commodity. Critics fear that holistic care is impossible if health services are defined in commodity terms for purchasing purposes, since purchasing tilts the scales toward those activities most easily measured: drug and surgical interventions, for example, rather than the less quantifiable nursing care. There is also concern that quality is less easily measured than cost. Does the race for greater efficiency lead to the risk of lower quality?

The blunt reality of health care is that a very small percentage of patients consumes the vast majority of care, as measured by cost. Paradoxically, those interventions that do the most good for the health status of the population, such as clean water and vaccinations, are relatively cost-effective and do not consume a significant portion of the health-care budget. For these reasons, no nation has chosen to supply health care on a purely market basis. Even the United States relies upon government programs like Medicaid and Medicare to cover the elderly and the poor, while leaving employers and individuals to shoulder the rest of the burden of coverage.

Regionalization and Devolution

Although Canada and the United States take quite different approaches to financing health care, the two countries' approaches to health-care service delivery are converging to some extent. In Canada, where government is the major single payer, provincial governments are devolving authority to regional or district entities that will manage demand for services in the context of their capped budgets.

In the United States, a new model of care provision, the integrated delivery network, is sparking interest in the management, not just of services, but also of demand. An individual episode of illness and its care have always been at the core of health-care approaches in both countries; now, however, a shift is under way as health policy planners increasingly think in terms of keeping people healthy throughout their lives, and improving the health of the population overall. As both the provider and payer side consolidate in the United States, it is becoming clear that lives will be "owned" and managed, in health-care terms, for longer periods of time. Therefore, service providers will have an incentive to manage those lives to an optimum health status so as to defer expensive treatment costs, or eliminate them altogether. On both sides of the border a new organizational form is emerging.

Another somewhat new idea taking hold in Canada is the regionalization of health services. By devolving authority to smaller-scale organizations, governments can achieve greater efficiency. On this principle, nine Canadian provinces have simultaneously pushed authority downward from their health ministries and pulled it upward from their hospital boards to concentrate it in a new entity: the regional health authority. While new to Canada, this practice has long been in place in the United Kingdom.

The early evidence from two of the first Canadian provinces to adopt this model, Alberta and Saskatchewan, is that the system works well in urban areas. Regional health authorities are meeting the goals set for them. Greater efficiency is being achieved. However, the regionalization of rural health services, which has been accompanied by the closure of many small hospitals, is less clearly a success. In small communities, cost savings from the closure of underused hospitals have not been reinvested in new delivery approaches.

From Inputs to Outcomes

Another idea that has gained extraordinary momentum in recent years in the health sector is that of evidence-based, or outcomes-based, practice. This idea is discussed in greater detail in Chapter 18.

For most of this century, our health-care delivery systems have been evaluated on the basis of inputs. We have measured the number of physicians, the number of dollars spent, the number of hospital beds. Growth in these inputs indicated a bigger, and therefore better, health-care system. Skepticism began to set in as it became apparent that health spending was reaching a point of diminishing returns. The 1980s and 1990s therefore saw the rise of the idea of evaluating medical and health interventions on the basis of outcomes rather than inputs.

Traditional health-care models considered evidence to be primarily a guide to whether or not a particular procedure or treatment was safe and potentially valuable. New approaches make much more use of evidence, focusing on statistically significant studies of what outcomes are achieved by particular interventions.

If new pharmaceutical interventions must be subject to randomized clinical trials, say the outcomes advocates, why not evaluate all medical interventions on the same basis? Why not ask, Does the surgery really work? Does the hospital stay extend life? Does the treatment alleviate pain? To what extent would a placebo work just as well? Is home care more effective for this condition? *How do we know?*

Many of the advocates of a greater focus on outcomes believe, based on evidence, that as much as 30% to 40% of what is done in the modern health-care system has no proven value. Practitioners argue back vehemently that much of what they do, even if its efficacy has not been scientifically demonstrated, is of value to the patient; that absence of proof is not to be taken as the inability to obtain proof; and that, in short, they would rather err on the side of conservatism — better to remove a few healthy appendixes than to risk an unnecessary death from a single diseased appendix.

Despite the persuasiveness of these counterarguments, the outcomes movement has grown rapidly, especially in the area of clinical epidemiology — the study of outcomes from clinical interventions, or, more often, the study of *patterns* of outcomes. Around the world, investments have been made by governments in this kind of health services research, and multinational efforts to share findings are gaining momentum.

Among the most significant investments in the outcomes movement is the British government's decision to allocate 1.5% of the National Health Service's total budget to health-services research (some £240 million per year). This effort, spearheaded by the dynamic Professor Michael Peckham, is a first step in shifting the entire basis of Britain's health system from history, politics, and tradition to evidence.

In the United States, the National Institutes of Health (the leading health research organizations funded by Washington) have also dedicated a portion of their budget to health-services research. Organizations such as the Rand Corporation, Kaiser Permanente's research centre, and many, many others have also begun to focus on outcomes-based research. The U.S. government established a research body, the Agency for Health Care Policy and Research a decade ago — though its funding was nearly cancelled by Congress after it produced findings on low back pain that were unpopular with the medical establishment. It survived this controversy, however, and over the past ten years the agency has progressed from methodological work to sponsoring the development of guidelines. It now sponsors systematic reviews of important clinical topics (the precursors of guidelines and quality improvement projects), as well as research on putting evidence-based findings into practice.

In Canada, the federal government and most provincial governments also support this new evidence-based effort to measure outcomes. Canada has created the Canadian Health Services Research Foundation. In the "austerity budget" of 1996, the foundation was the only new spending initiative. Other organizations that sponsor research into the actual outcomes of particular health or medical interventions have sprung up across the country, such as the Manitoba Centre for Health Policy and Evaluation, the Institute for Clinical Evaluative Sciences, and the Saskatchewan Utilization Management Commission. Already, some intriguing findings have been reported:

◇ Home care is a cost-effective alternative to much hospital care (Saskatchewan Utilization Management Commission).
◇ An aspirin a day taken after a first heart attack dramatically reduces the occurrence of second heart attacks (Institute for Clinical Evaluative Sciences study).
◇ Some 85% of emergency-ward ankle X-rays are unnecessary (University of Ottawa study with Institute for Clinical Evaluative Sciences).
◇ Low-back pain is readily treated by massage therapists and chiropractors as well as by physicians (Agency for Healthcare Research and Quality).

◇ Hospital bed closures do not necessarily decrease quality of care (Manitoba Centre for Health Policy and Evaluation).

The World Bank devoted its annual report in 1993 to the issue of health and evidence. (The importance placed on this issue by a bank — an institution not usually associated with health care — is another indication of the impact of broader determinants of health.) The evidence-based approach is central to the current work of the World Bank, which chooses health interventions on the basis of a measurement called the DALY: disability-adjusted life years. If, for example, spending $1 million (U.S.) on a vaccination program will add twice as many DALYs as spending the same $1 million on cardiac bypass surgery, the bank will support vaccination, to achieve the greatest good for the greatest number.

The application of utilitarianism to health systems is not new, of course. The innovation in outcomes-based health policy consists in the explicit measurement of particular interventions and corresponding quantitative calculations of their utility. This approach has affected not only the adoption of new interventions in health-care systems around the world, but has caused a rethinking of some existing interventions in terms of their actual efficacy and cost-effectiveness.

Conclusions

A broader definition of health; integration of care; regionalization; a market approach to purchasing — together, these powerful new ideas are a major force for change in health care as we enter the twenty-first century, the first of the four winds blowing our societies in new directions. While many of these new ideas may seem obvious to an observer from outside the health sector, from within they may seem both exhilarating and, at times, threatening. The culture of health care is conservative, and the notion that a venerable hospital must suddenly learn to negotiate with a purchaser demanding a better deal, or that a world-class medical centre may be pushed into insolvency if it fails to react quickly to newly unleashed market forces, can be profoundly disturbing. And evidence-based practice can lead to some approaches that are quite fundamentally different to those we have long followed in our pursuit of better ways of treating illness. Yet the seeds blown in on the wind of these new ideas will grow into the health systems of tomorrow.

Another reason to be cautious is the fact that the health sector is unique. Unlike many other services we seek, we are likely to need health care only infrequently during our lifetimes. But at those moments when we are faced with an acute or critical illness, our very survival may depend on the correct intervention. That intervention may be rather modest, like the taking of an antibiotic drug, or it may be quite major, like the treatment of a series of traumatic injuries from an automobile accident. As individuals, we cannot predict which health services we will need or what they will cost. Some of us may need a treatment that exceeds our annual earnings, or even our lifetime earnings. This is why most systems have some element of sharing risk, either socializing costs through the state or pooling the risk through private insurance.

Providers often complain that reformers are ill-informed about the reality of care delivery. This is true. The powerful ideas discussed here are just that: ideas. Their roots are intellectual and their merits can be judged only after their application to the real world. In some cases, those in the field have been pleasantly surprised by the practical benefits of some new thinking. GP fundholding in the United Kingdom fits this category. Other ideas, such as the Crown health enterprises in New Zealand, turn out not to achieve their promise in the real-world laboratory of practice. We must be wary of "idea tourism," of change purely for the sake of change. As Professor Ted Marmor of the Yale School of Management has accurately pointed out, bad ideas travel just as readily as good ones.

Health systems at the turn of the millennium are being shaped by powerful forces. Politicians, policy makers, and health managers must respond by drawing upon powerful concepts. Often these concepts are compelling as theory but challenging to implement. Trial and error forms a critical element of the learning process. New concepts must be hoisted on the mast of the health-care delivery vessel, where they will either fly proudly or be torn apart by the winds of change.

2

•

New Public Expectations:
Quality, Speed, and Appropriateness

*U.K. patients and the public are grossly uninformed — depen-
dants, not partners in health care. . . . They judge quality by access
to hospital services.*
— JENNY GRIFFITHS, U.K. HEALTH PURCHASING EXECUTIVE (1996)

Around the world, users of health care in developed nations are thinking less like recipients and more like consumers. In places like Canada
and the United Kingdom, fifty years of the welfare state have left an
indelible imprint on health-care users, but their attitude is slowly changing. The degree and nature of this revolution varies markedly by nation.
Nevertheless, it is essentially a worldwide revolution. Attitudes and
expectations are rapidly and markedly transforming as health consumers
are becoming more educated and more demanding.

This revolution among health-care consumers takes several forms. In many countries where health-care services have been an endeavour in the public sector, it manifests itself as a movement away from a "one size fits all" model and toward a network of much more individualized services and greater consumer choice. In the United States, consumers are challenging "closed-panel" health maintenance organizations that restrict their clients' access to a limited list of physicians. In Canada and the United Kingdom, health ministers are constantly questioned about the long waiting lists for certain procedures. In South Africa, the Nelson Mandela government wrestled with the demand from black South Africans for quality health services.

But in every nation, consumers' demands are ultimately similar. They want quality, speed, choice, appropriateness of care, and affordability.

Quality

Public opinion about health care is undergoing a major shift. Thirty years ago, people simply wanted access to health services. Today, a more savvy public wants quality, too.

As a student at Harvard in the early 1970s, I toured the great, old General Motors plant in Framingham, Massachusetts. At the end of the assembly line, massive auto workers were hammering the doors of Cadillacs with huge rubber mallets; only after serious pounding did the doors fit. When I asked our tour guide what the workers were doing, she said simply, "Quality control." In those earlier consumer days, quality was an add-on, applied by a big rubber mallet after the fact. Later, faced with stiff competition from the Japanese and German car industries, North American auto makers began a necessary shift to engineering quality into the product during the manufacturing process. Quality became "Job 1" at Ford.

Similarly, quality control in medicine and health services has too often been considered only after the fact — often in the form of a coroner's inquest, or a lawsuit from a grieving parent. Only in the last few years has this same consumer pressure for quality come fully to bear on the health-care delivery system. Quality has to become Job 1 in health care; consumers will settle for no less.

For many people, choice is a necessary prerequisite for quality. In the old days, patients were happy that there was a doctor in place, a hospital open nearby, and a nurse present. Now patients demand options; they want to participate in selecting a surgeon or family practitioner. And once they have settled on one, they are not nearly as willing to take his or her word that everything is okay. Growing up, I thought it was a miracle that we had one channel on our black-and-white TV. Later, when we got five or six channels, and then a colour TV, I considered it a vast improvement. Now everyone I know has fifty channels and a large-screen colour TV with stereo sound. If we don't like a program, we just click through it. The children demand to know, "When we are getting 200 channels? Why is the Internet access so slow?" Like this new generation of television viewers, today's health-care consumer holds the remote control ever at the ready.

The public resists the idea that one size fits all. People want health care that meets needs of varying kinds. I remember seeing, for a long time, a sign on a construction site near my home that read "Health Clinic Coming." I kept watching to see who the doctors would be. When the clinic opened, I discovered that its occupants were an aromatherapist, three kinds of massage therapists, and an occupational therapist — not a single doctor. Yet the building is undeniably a health clinic.

Speed

In most service industries, speed is one standard by which service is measured. In Canadian urban centres, Pizza Pizza delivers in thirty minutes or the pizza is free. FedEx promises to deliver your package by 10:30 a.m. the next day. These service standards for speed have two qualities: first, they are explicit, and hence can be evaluated by the consumer. Second, there are penalties for failure to perform — specific penalties, clearly understood by both seller and consumer, that require no review committees or courts to implement. If the pizza doesn't arrive, then Pizza Pizza has failed to perform and so pays an immediate price. The pizza is free.

Our society's obsession with speed has spread to other service industries: hotels offer one-minute check-in at the desk — not to mention check-out from right in the room. Airlines offer electronic tickets that are "issued" the minute you book the flight and picked up in moments at the airport counter. All across the service sector, the silicon chip has been used to reduce or eliminate lineups and otherwise increase the pace at which services can be delivered. Speed with measurable, consumer-transparent standards has become a requirement for customer satisfaction.

One excellent example of the consumer quest for speed and quality in health services is the explosive growth of laser eye surgery. Chains of clinics offering this service, where consumers gladly pay $1,000 to $4,000 (U.S.) to have their eyes reshaped and their vision improved, have rapidly appeared across North America. A key aspect of their business is speed. This is a health service measured in minutes, not weeks or months. The ten-minute "eye job" is the most rapidly growing medical procedure today.

One example of how this concept has affected the health-care system is the revolution in the speed with which new treatments, particularly new drugs, now enter into widespread use. Advocacy by HIV/AIDS patients has led the way in this area, encouraging other patient groups to campaign for much more rapid approvals of new treatments. The U.S. regulatory agency, the Federal Drug Administration (FDA), has been under enormous political pressure to speed up its reviews, and to some extent it has responded. Other nations have also seen lobbying for accelerated reviews.

There are, however, risks associated with a more rapid approval process. If all the consequences of a new medical product are not understood before it is used widely, a disaster is possible. In the consumer's mind, speed does not justify the sacrifice of quality. Just as a pizza delivered in thirty minutes is not acceptable if it is cold or burnt, day surgery must be faster than a hospital stay but provide an equally good recovery.

If our health-care system sacrifices quality for speed it will be as popular as a cold pizza — and much more dangerous.

Appropriateness

To the issues of speed and quality we can add a third major new public expectation: care must be appropriate. A fast, competently executed, but wholly unnecessary Caesarean section or hysterectomy is not acceptable to today's pregnant woman. Patients want to be confident that their treatment is relevant to their specific case, not based on historic custom or a new medical fad.

Studies show that the rate at which certain procedures are performed vary widely, and that the differences are based more on geography than on differences in medical need. This kind of information troubles patients. As health consumers become more informed about these issues, they are less inclined to consider doctors the only infallible judges of the appropriateness of a procedure or treatment. Where once we held our health-care providers in the highest regard, we now increasingly question their authority. Our doctors are no longer on pedestals; they have fallen from a great height.

Consumer Supremacy

Harvard Business School Professor Regina Herzlinger begins her important book *Market Driven Health Care* by asking why Toyota repair rates are easier to find than heart surgeon survival rates. Ms. Herzlinger argues that what she calls "consumer supremacy" is "the key to the successful transformation of the retailing, automobile, and information industries," and goes on to consider whether it might similarly reinvent the American health-care sector: "Can Americans obtain better and lower-cost health care? . . . The answer is a resounding Yes." The consumer revolution, in her view, is like an earthquake that will shake up the current, failing, badly organized model.

Professor Herzlinger advocates a "consumer-controlled health system," which, she suggests, will foster innovation. Yet despite the passion of her advocacy, she is brought up somewhat short by the current realities of the American health system. Consumers are not, directly, payers; most health bills are paid by employers or by governments. In the end, she can only advocate that consumers be more determined and vigilant, and that payees and governments empower patients with information rather than strangling them with rules. This is solid advice, but until U.S. consumers have real choice over their providers, the predicted earthquake may turn out to be little more than a tremor in that country.

Meanwhile, over in Europe, Franz Knieps, director of Health Policy for the German Federal Association of Regional Sickness Funds, in a 1998 paper, has commented on the consumer in the context of Germany thus:

> Consumers' needs and choices will design the health-care system of the future. Equal access, transparency, high quality, speed (no waiting lists), effectiveness, effectivity, and efficiency will be the parameter of integrated care. Institutional interests and personal incomes must consider the winds of change — otherwise the German health care will be shaken fundamentally.

Even the German health system, which has traditionally been marked by stability — its roots were established in the time of Otto von Bismarck, "the Iron Chancellor," a century and a half ago — is due to be reshaped by the consumer.

Conclusions

Public expectations will profoundly alter many of the old realities of health-care delivery. The most educated generation in the history of our species will not meekly accept the status quo. Change is certain. A large cohort of informed, demanding consumers are entering the fifty-plus age range. As the health-care needs of the boomer generation increase (despite their health foods, vitamins, and Nikes), so will their demands for speed, quality, and appropriateness in health care.

This desire to have a say in their health-care system is deeply felt by the public today. One cross-national study, titled *The Cost of Health System Change* (Donelan et al., 1999), found that health-care experiences and major policy changes that affect them are "central to individual and family security." In all five countries surveyed (Australia, Canada, New Zealand, the United Kingdom, and the United States), "[e]xposure to high out-of-pocket costs, difficulties obtaining care, and fears that quality of care is declining prompt[ed] widespread public dissatisfaction. . . . As countries grapple with how to improve their citizens' health and quality of life while trying to use more efficient health-care resources, popular perceptions of the impact of change are likely to be of increasing importance, particularly in the realm of politics and elections." Therefore, the study's authors concluded, "Policy makers in all nations need to understand that the public notices the impact of policy changes in health care and frequently bears new and unexpected costs or barriers to care unwillingly."

3

•

Technology:
Chip-Driven Change

The number of transistors on a silicon chip seems to double every
year.

— GORDON MOORE, CHAIR EMERITUS, INTEL (1965)

Perhaps the strongest of the winds driving change in health-delivery
systems worldwide is the technological revolution. The new millennium
will witness wave upon wave of health innovation — remarkable drugs,
gene therapies, new vaccines, and miraculous nanomachines that travel
within the human body. They will stretch our imagination and challenge our ethical foundations and values. The ubiquitous silicon chip,
which has transformed our ability to obtain, store, and manage information, is profoundly affecting health-care delivery in a myriad of ways.

Other important technological advances include great strides in biotechnology and a move toward miniaturization.

Chip-driven computer technology has also led to a transformation of the big picture, providing us with powerful tools for discovering patterns of health and illness, and for charting the complex outcomes of particular health-care interventions. Information drives change. The silicon chip, as a tool for managing information, is actually transforming how we think about health and illness. It is also changing how we organize, manage, and deliver health services.

The better we can measure, the better we must manage. So long as measurement lagged, health care remained a fragmented and unaccountable industry. Moore's Law (the Intel chair later revised his estimate of the time it takes for chip capacity to double to a whopping eighteen months) is unlikely to be repealed anytime soon.

Just as the silicon chip and the power of information technology have transformed other sectors, from finance to communication, so too they are beginning to transform health care, though in less obvious ways. There is no single piece of technology that has affected health care the way the ATM has transformed banking. There is not a single consumer device, such as the personal computer, to symbolize the transformation. Nevertheless, health care–related applications for silicon chips abound, from sophisticated imaging machines to electronic record-management systems, to handheld monitors that allow doctors to do lab tests at the bedside, to sophisticated telecommunications devices that save massive amounts of time and labour. Recent advances in computing, furthermore, have given researchers the ability to manipulate large quantities of data relating to treatments and outcomes, without which the evidence-based revolution discussed in Chapter 1 would be impossible.

Speed, Speed!

An astonishing feature of the digital age is the speed with which new technologies are now diffused. As the following table shows, it took thirty-seven years for the first 10 million telephones to enter use. The cell phone required only eight years to reach its first 10 million customers. Compare that to the mere six months for 10 million Web browsers to be up and running. The future in which Internet access is as widespread as the telephone or television is very near indeed.

Years to 10 Million Users

Technology	Years from Introduction to 10 Million Users
Pager	40
Telephone	37
Cable TV	24
Fax	21
VCR	10
Cell phone	8
PC	6
CD ROM	5
Web browser	0.5

Source: Morgan Stanley Technology Research, 1999.

Cost Savings

Why are ATMs so popular with the public? They are convenient, easy to use, and reliable. Why are ATMs popular with the banks? They are economical. The cost of a bank transaction involving a human teller is roughly $2.00 (CDN). By contrast, an ATM-based transaction costs on average $0.06. Thus, a bank can process thirty-three transactions at an ATM for the same cost as one teller-based transaction.

Similarly, chip-driven technology is being applied to the high-cost transactions of the health-care world. While working at the Ontario Ministry of Health, I learned that processing a paper claim from a doctor cost roughly $0.25 (CDN) more than processing a machine-readable claim. By adding a fee to paper claims, the ministry encouraged doctors to convert to the machine-readable format, saving taxpayers about $25 million on the more than 100 million claims made in the province per year. Imagine applying similar cost efficiencies to each of the tens of billions of health-care transactions made in North America per year — not to mention the associated potential improvements in speed and accuracy.

Less Invasive Diagnosis and Treatment Options

Diagnostic imaging — all those fancy machines with acronyms like CTs, MRIs, and PETs — are really silicon chips, too, in an elaborate package. Driven by computing power and able to provide images of the insides of the human body, these new imaging technologies are transforming the diagnosis of illness. Exploratory surgery, in many parts of the human anatomy, has given way to exploratory imaging. Surgeons can now see accurately inside joints, hearts, and even brains without raising their scalpels.

My late father, Percy, an orthopedic surgeon, prepared on Sunday evenings for his Monday surgeries. As a young boy I would sit with him in his study as he examined the shadowy X-rays on which his surgery would be based. He would be astonished if he could see the clear, photograph-quality images of the inside of a knee joint or a hip that doctors now have access to, just twenty years after his death. Underlying all these new technologies is the ability of silicon chips to translate electrons into accurate images.

Diagnostic imaging allows a doctor less invasive and, often, more accurate ways of finding out what's wrong; but of course, technology has also revolutionized the way physicians *treat* a number of problems as well. While imaging machines get bigger, many other advances depend on technology getting smaller. Tiny machines and tools are allowing new surgical procedures that reduce trauma to the body and shorten recovery times. Minuscule cameras can go down arteries; using minimally invasive surgery, also called laparoscopy, surgeons can do through tiny incisions what once required a large opening. Laparoscopy rates are climbing steadily, and have reached over 90% for gallbladder operations and over 70% for gynecology procedures. This ability of surgeons to perform major procedures, such as heart bypass operations, through very small openings, depends on new, smaller tools and the use of fibre optics.

New Communication Tools

The telecommunications revolution of cell phones, pagers, and call centres is also based in silicon. When I visited the Access Health call centre in Sacramento, California, the feature that struck me as most remarkable was the set of computers that supported the nurses assisting patients. The ability of the software to translate answers to simple questions — Are you dizzy? Are you bleeding? — into clinical frame-works was impressive. These computer-based protocols did not replace a nurse's judgment, but rather complemented and reinforced it: the ubiq-uitous chip making its presence felt in yet another health-delivery role.

Another communications-related consequence of the supremacy of the chip is the potential for "unbundling" the delivery of health infor-mation from the patient's visit. Traditional health systems pay for each provider/patient encounter: a visit to a physician's office, a house call, an encounter with a health professional in a nursing home, a lab test, or an actual surgical procedure. Many of these encounters are initiated by patients seeking information, not care, in the first instance. Nurse call lines and Internet-based health-information services reduce the need for these information-seeking visits. Often second visits are to obtain results, which could also often be given over the phone. In these days when we pay bills, book plane tickets, and basically run our lives by phone, why must we always see a doctor face to face? The Ontario Medical Association has been pushing for physicians to bill for time spent on the phone. Technology has also speeded up diagnostic testing and detached it from the necessity of a doctor's visit.

The separation of communicating health information and clinical insight from the physical encounter of the patient is the underpinning for radical changes in the location and nature of care.

An Explosion of Information

A recent report titled *A New Perspective on Health Policy* (Glouberman et al., 1999) describes the information explosion in health care thus: "One thing that has undeniably changed during the past twenty-five years is that there has been an explosion of available health data, resulting from increased computing power, statistical sophistication, and more comprehensive survey instruments, which collectively allow for detailed analysis of population health indicators. . . ."

There are certainly better, more thorough databases in the health field (and indeed in all fields) today than there were a generation ago. One sign of the explosion of information we have seen since the beginning of the Lalonde era is the vastly increased number of professional publications in the life sciences. From 1975 to the end of the century, the number of professional scientific journals in the field of genetics alone increased from 61 to 256, and in the field of neuroscience from 45 to 473.

And not only is more raw empirical data available, but there have been many innovations in the collation, storage, and distribution of this information involving the new technologies of recent years, such as easy-to-use spreadsheet and statistical applications software, and nearly universal access to affordable computers that can run this software.

Also crucial to the impact of the information explosion on the health systems of the world are organizations that facilitate the distribution of all this new knowledge, such as the Cochrane Collaboration (see Chapter 18 for details). And, of course, the Internet and its databases and search engines (such as OVID and Medline) put data that was once found only on major university library shelves into easy reach of anyone with a modem.

Finding It in Cyberspace

In fact, the influence of the Internet on the ease of access an ordinary, middle-class resident of the Western world has to health-related information has already been huge, and has the potential to expand much further. In just one recent month, for example (July 1999), the nine top health Internet sites attracted more than a million different visitors each.

Top Ten Internet Health Sites

Web Site	Millions of Visitors in July 1999
drkoop.com	1.397
Third Age	1.354
Health Shop	1.327
NIH.gov	1.231
PlanetRx	1.171
Mother Nature	1.163
On Health	1.142
Thrive Online	1.012
Drugstore.com	1.006

Source: Wit Capital, *Wit's Wisdom on eHealth*, September 20, 1999.

From January to July 1999, the number of people in North America using the Internet for reasons related to health information increased from 23 million to 70 million. The top site alone, drkoop.com, reported that its traffic increased by 58% between July and August of 1999.

Clearly, the Web will be a major force in twenty-first-century health care. Health Canada, for example, has recently entered this ring as well with a publicly accessible set of documents on all aspects of health, including recent research reports, on its Web site. But the Internet is most likely to affect patients in their roles as consumers. By providing consumers with access to a vast reservoir of information, it will shift power from providers to users. It will also support doctors, nurses, and pharmacists in providing better services to patients.

Strides in Information Processing

The current proliferation of available data would be of little use without the means to process and analyze it. Fortunately, this explosion of information comes at precisely a time when we have the computing power to make use of it — not, of course, coincidentally, since the information explosion has itself, in part, been fuelled by developments in computer technology.

The *New Perspective* study details the effect of these developments on health care as follows:

When the data for the Lalonde report was being collected, computers occupied whole buildings, operating on stacks of punch cards, carrying out lists of simple instructions, albeit with amazing speed and accuracy for the time. They were not only large and slow but also expensive — beyond the means of any but the largest corporations and educational institutions. Today's supercomputers have processing speeds of approximately 1,000 billion instructions per second. And while supercomputers are still beyond the means of most users, even the most underfunded research lab now has desktop computers that far exceed the capacity of the major research computers of the Lalonde era.

Hand in hand with the developments of computer technology have been a number of developments in statistical methodology. There have been some genuine innovations in statistical practice in the past twenty-five years, but perhaps more important than these is the fact that a number of older, yet powerful, techniques that were once seldom employed because of the vast amounts of computation they required have now come into widespread use.

The birth of the new information age is one of the forces that will determine the eventual shape of health policy in this century. Never before in human history has there been the potential to create, manipulate, analyze, and distribute so much information; this phenomenon is revolutionizing all fields, including health.

Mapping the Human Genome

No discussion of the impact of new technology on health would be complete without mention of the big event in biomedical research: the Human Genome Project, which has as its goal nothing short of mapping the 80,000 genes within human DNA. The science of gene sequencing, or mapping, is one that could hardly even have been conceived of a generation ago, yet, today, advances in microscopy and computing, and in laboratory techniques that allow us to amplify minute quantities of a specific gene and determine its entire sequence at the same time, have made it one of the most vital and important areas of medical research. Once all our genetic building blocks are revealed, the potential for developing new treatments based on this expanded understanding is immense.

DNA and genes are the centre of an enormous, worldwide biotechnology revolution. This field is expanding rapidly, not only because of endeavours like the Human Genome Project, but also because of research related to such diverse organisms as bacteria, animals, and plants. Research companies and scientists in universities are pursuing the next new thing — complete knowledge of the detailed structure of life itself.

New genes are now discovered on a weekly basis. These genes are sometimes linked to human disease, and when this is the case, often as rapidly as the genes are discovered, a new diagnostic-testing technique related to the associated disease is developed. Gene therapies to ultimately treat the disease are also investigated.

All these complex technologies are dependent on our ability to manipulate DNA, the nucleic acid in each of your body's cells that carries your genetic information. DNA is coiled up in packages called chromosomes. Every normal human being has forty-six of these chromosomes — twenty-three from each of your parents.

Your genes — you have more than 50,000 of them — are contained in the chromosomes. You can think of a gene as a specific section of a chromosome, or as a stretch of DNA. The fundamental set of genes that defines an organism is called the genome, and the goal of decoding the complete human genome is such an exciting one that an actual race is now under way.

The prestigious U.S. National Institutes of Health (the leading centre for health research in the world), along with the U.S. Department of

Energy, launched the $3 billion (U.S.) Human Genome Project in 1995, with a plan to sequence the full genome by 2005. In mid-1998, scientist and entrepreneur Dr. J. Craig Venter announced a competing private-sector initiative with an ambitious three-year time schedule. No overall winner has yet been declared in this fascinating race between traditional public sector–financed research and private-sector entrepreneurial dynamism. However, the Venter initiative is on schedule and appears to have the potential to succeed. Both groups now deny that there is a contest and argue that they are advancing science cooperatively.

Conclusions

The technology drivers are powerful. First, the silicon chip has ushered in the digital revolution in health. *Everything* will be measured and hence, eventually, managed. Next the genome revolution will utterly tranform our approach to health care. By allowing treatment of health conditions previously considered untreatable, gene therapy will profoundly change some people's lives. As well, because we will all gain insight into our genetic makeup and health risks, we will all be made more aware of our mortality and fragility.

In the face of all this technological change with its undeniable advantages, we would do well to remember a caution from poet T.S. Eliot in "The Rock," which he penned with canny foresight well before the computing age: "Where is the wisdom we have lost in knowledge? Where is the knowledge we have lost in information?" Science, technology, and information must be complementary to wisdom in our society, not substitutes for it.

4

•

Fiscal Constraints:
The Big Squeeze

*Paradoxically, the effort to better contain costs has led to more
effective health care with better outcomes.*
— OECD, *BETTER HEALTH AT LOWER COST?* (JUNE 23, 1998)

When prime ministers and presidents advocate more cost-effective
health services, their thinking has been profoundly shaped by a mild-
mannered Belgian statistician whom they have never met. Jean-Pierre
Poullier toiled for many years at the Organisation for Economic Co-oper-
ation and Development (OECD), that "club" of the industrialized
nations, headquartered in Paris. Poullier's enormous contribution was to
measure health spending, nation by nation. The exhaustive reconcilia-
tion of different categories of health expenditures was the key challenge
in this task; each nation counts its health spending in a different

manner. Yet thanks to Poullier's measurements, the ratio of health spending to gross national product (GNP) has become the most widely used method for international comparisons of health spending. The leaders of nations worldwide use this measure when judging their own spending policies in the area of health.

For 1996, the OECD countries devoted, on average, 8.2% of their GNPs to health spending. This total includes both public- and private-sector spending. The range of spending levels among the nations is significant:

Top Five Spenders on Health Care in OECD

Country	Share of Gross National Product Spent on Health Care, 1996
United States	14.0%
Germany	10.5%
Switzerland	10.2%
France	9.7%
Canada	9.6%

Source: OECD Health Data 1998, Paris.

The lowest levels, not surprisingly, occurred in some of the poorer OECD countries:

Bottom Five Spenders on Health Care in OECD

Country	Share of Gross National Product Spent on Health Care, 1996
Hungary	6.7%
Poland	5.0%
Mexico	4.6%
Korea	4.0%
Turkey	3.8%

Source: OECD Health Data 1998, Paris.

Because of vast differences in income levels across nations, the differences in per capita spending are even greater. The United States spent $3,898 (U.S.) for each man, woman, and child on health care in 1996, versus a mere $232 (U.S.) in Turkey, $371 (U.S.) in Poland, and $358 (U.S.) in Mexico.

The notion of comparing health outcomes to spending has become a major political focus, thanks to M. Poullier's numbers. For example, despite low levels of spending, Mexico experienced a drop of over 70% in its premature mortality rate, which is defined as the number of years of life lost before age seventy that are considered to be preventable. This impressive improvement was a result of such factors as medical advances, better social amenities, a cleaner environment, and healthier lifestyles.

This absence of a direct correlation between spending and outcomes laid the groundwork for health-cost-containment thinking. This idea most particularly has caught the attention of the United States, which is the outlier in terms of spending a great deal more than other nations without apparent benefit in terms of reducing avoidable deaths.

While M. Poullier has been counting, another astute observer of global health development, Robert Maxwell, the former chief executive of the London-based King's Fund, has taken on the task of describing the broad sweep of postwar health policies across the industrialized world.

His findings are summarized in the table below.

Postwar Health Policies of Industrialized Nations

Era	Salient Features of National Health Policies
1945 to 1975	• rebuilding • extending coverage • improving services incrementally • emphasis on public finance
1975 to 1990	• caps on public expenditure • increased supply-side efficiency • renewed interest in supplementing public financing

Postwar Health Policies of Industrialized Nations (cont'd)

Era	Salient Features of National Health Policies
1990 and on	• obtaining value within public sector • managing demand as well as supply • managing public/private mix

Source: Dr. Robert J. Maxwell, "Beyond Restructuring: The Limit of Simple Fixes."
Presentation to the OHA convention, Toronto, November 4, 1997.

1945 to 1975: The Spending Boom

In the postwar era — the 1950s, 1960s, and early 1970s in most industrialized nations — dollars flowed to health care with few barriers. This was the era of building, coincident with the baby boom. Nations built and rebuilt facilities for an entire generation of doctors, nurses, and other health-care professionals. Bigger was better: three cars in the driveway, new wings on the hospital, more of everything. Health care would give us immortality. Social policy wars were launched: in the United States, President Nixon declared a war on cancer, and President Johnson a war on poverty. Health-care services began to consume more and more of the resources of society. It was not until the late 1970s that some questioning began of how these dollars were being spent.

This spending boom represents one of the great investments in health in the history of our species. What compelled us to invest so many resources in health care at this time?

The major factors were buoyant economies and the postwar baby boom. Accommodating this boom, as well as the rise of many new medical techniques, accounted for much of the spending explosion. The rise of the U.S. manufacturing economy, with its high-wage blue-collar jobs complete with generous health benefits, also fuelled the expansion of the health-care sector. Among employers in the United States and governments in Canada alike, the most popular spending program quickly became health services.

1975 to 1990: Spending Caps and Supply-Side Management

In the last quarter of the century, growth in health spending began to slow. From 2.5% of GDP in 1960, it had been growing rapidly, then more sedately, to reach 5.4 % of GDP by 1980. Average annual growth across the OECD nations went down to 3.9% in 1976–82, then to 3.6% in 1983–89.

What led to this squeezing of health spending? First, the public sector was facing unsustainable deficits in many jurisdictions, and the private sector was feeling pressures on profits. About the same time in the late 1980s that many in corporate America discovered that employee health costs had exceeded their total profits, government leaders in some countries and provinces discovered that health spending exceeded their total deficits. As economic growth slowed, the funding of growth in health spending came to depend on borrowed money.

Here in Canada, as the table below shows, growth in total health expenditure peaked in 1981–82, the middle of Maxwell's second era, then began to slow substantially. On average during the 1976–1989 period, it grew at an annual rate of 11.6%.

Total Annual Health-Care Spending in Canada, 1975–1989

Year	Millions of $	% Growth	% of GNP
1975	12,260.1	—	7.1
1976	14,102.5	15.0	7.0
1977	15,500.9	9.9	7.0
1978	17,172.1	10.8	7.0
1979	19,230.8	12.0	6.9
1980	22,371.9	16.3	7.1
1981	26,386.2	17.9	7.3
1982	30,914.4	17.2	8.1
1983	34,190.9	10.6	8.3
1984	36,870.0	7.8	8.2
1985	39,985.8	8.5	8.2

**Total Annual Health-Care Spending
in Canada, 1975–1989 (cont'd)**

Year	Millions of $	% Growth	% of GNP
1986	43,499.8	8.8	8.5
1987	46,980.6	8.0	8.4
1988	51,154.9	8.9	8.4
1989	56,366.4	10.2	8.6

Source: Canadian Institute for Health Information, *National Health Expenditures*, 1999.

The 1990s: Obtaining Value

The 1990s continued the fiscal squeeze across OECD countries, and Canada was no exception. Between 1991 and 1996, the average annual rate of growth was only 2.5%. Expenditures reached $77.1 billion (CDN) in 1997 and $80.0 billion in 1998, representing a slight increase in the growth rate to 3.8%.

Another way of viewing the rise and subsequent fall in health-care spending growth is to examine the share of GNP devoted to health services. In the table below, note the rise from 7.0% of GNP in 1976–78 to a peak of 10% in 1992. Note also the decline to 8.9% by 1997.

As we enter the new millennium health spending is once again rising but more slowly than it did in the 1970s and 1980s. A lively debate is now under way among those who advocate more spending and those who favour efficiencies.

Total Annual Health-Care Spending in Canada, 1990–1999

Year	Millions of $	% Growth	% of GNP
1990	61,305.7	8.8	9.0
1991	66,529.7	8.5	9.7
1992	70,061.6	5.3	10.0
1993	71,972.6	2.7	9.9
1994	73,578.9	2.2	9.6

Total Annual Health-Care Spending
in Canada, 1990–1999 (cont'd)

Year	Millions of $	% Growth	% of GNP
1995	74,616.5	1.4	9.2
1996	75,601.9	1.3	9.1
1997	77,955.5	3.1	8.9
1998*	81,822.3	5.0	9.1
1999*	86,013.1	5.1	9.2

* = forecast

Source: Canadian Institute for Health Information, *National Health Expenditures*, 1999.

Techniques for reducing spending changed in the 1990s from broad supply-side constraints to reengineering care delivery in search of better value for the health-care dollar. My own career in government provided me with a ringside seat for health-spending decisions. In the early 1970s, as a young public servant in Manitoba, I participated in the annual budget process. The Health Minister carried the largest stick at the Cabinet table. His colleagues believed that health spending was essential to political popularity, even to political survival. They governed themselves accordingly and approved large increases in health spending.

By the mid-1980s, the overall financial pressures on the treasury caused at least the Finance Minister to question health spending more closely. By the early 1990s, when I was Deputy Minister of Health in Ontario, my minister and I faced a Cabinet skeptical of the benefits of increased health spending. Each year, in fact, reductions were sought, and it became conventional wisdom that efficiencies were possible in health services.

The early initiatives were supply-side constraints: reductions to hospital budgets, tougher negotiations with doctors, nurses, and pharmacists, and reductions to medical-school enrollments. By the mid-1990s, a general restructuring of health services was moving rapidly forward, driven by financial imperatives. In the late 1990s, initiatives began to focus on the demand side of the equation. Efforts to introduce health call centres, better health information, a renewal of public health initiatives, and the emergence of population health were all indications of these changes.

A comparison of the challenges faced by health policy makers across a number of nations turns up more similarities than differences; Canada's experience paralleled that of the other industrialized countries. After two decades of health spending growing faster than inflation, and much faster than population growth, the music — and the funding — stopped. Health services met the fiscal wall. In most nations the growth of health spending slowed dramatically. In some subnational jurisdictions, actual reductions in total health spending occurred.

Franz Knieps, an astute observer of the German health scene, has described how this phenomenon played out in the employer-financed German sickness funds as follows:

The German health-care system is working under a growing financial and political pressure driven by global forces. Unemployment and burden shifting from pension funds and unemployment insurance to sickness funds lead to stagnation of the funds' resources. Employers and employees will not accept rising contribution rates any more, especially as long as rising premiums lead to rising co-payments. So cost containment will go on after general elections this year [1998].

Health policy is shifting from preserving traditional structures towards integrated care which takes responsibility for management of costs and quality. Aspects of public health are becoming more important than individual interests of providers and consumers. Public money will be spent mainly for public goods.

In each nation, the health-spending boom has given way to capping and, later, to a search for better value in return for existing levels of spending.

Conclusions

Despite the big squeeze applied to health-care spending in recent years, the OECD recently concluded that "the state of health of populations in the twenty-nine Member countries of the OECD continues to improve, and expenditure on health as a share of GNP has stabilized somewhat on the whole after a decade or more of health-care reform in many OECD countries."

While the slowing of growth in health spending is often blamed for much of the current stress felt by both providers and patients, this fiscal imperative in fact has sparked massive and necessary reforms. Financial pressure served as the catalyst to a rethinking of our priorities in health. It also shook many cherished beliefs in health care, causing a "stampede among the many sacred cows," as one Canadian health economist observed, reviewing the debates of the mid-1990s. No longer was questioning health-related spending — or health professionals, for that matter — unthinkable. As Robert Maxwell noted, the era of obtaining value within the public sector began in the early 1990s, and continues unabated today.

Funding constraints have their largest impact on the timing of change, not its direction. The other three winds are shaping where we are going; the big squeeze on dollars shapes when we go there. The financial pressures leading governments and employers to dramatically reduce the growth of spending on health services have sparked a restructuring of health-care delivery, but many aspects of this have been profoundly shaped by the other forces of change discussed in earlier chapters. New technologies and drugs, for example, have made shorter hospital stays medically possible; financial pressures have dictated when we implemented these shorter stays as general policy.

The big financial squeeze is a major event in the evolution of health-care service delivery. Although the squeezing has now abated somewhat, no return to double-digit spending growth in OECD countries is forecast. Health-care reform needed a "burning platform" to compel movement away from a tenacious status quo; funding cutbacks provided both the gasoline and the spark. They also absorbed all of the blame from providers for the often painful transformation of long-standing practices and approaches to care. The mantra of government leaders and health managers became "We *must* change how we care for people because we simply do not have the money to continue as we have done."

There is no consensus regarding the long-term results of the big squeeze. The OECD and many other observers hold the view that the overall impact was a positive one: better outcomes at lower cost, a bargain for taxpayers and employers. Most providers, not surprisingly, hold the opposing view. Nurses who saw their jobs disappear by the thousands from hospitals are convinced that the recent cutbacks hurt not only them but their patients. Physicians, whose incomes have felt the squeeze (or at minimum a modest pinch) share this view. No one disputes the power of fiscal constraints to motivate change; the disagreement is about the consequences of the changes.

For my part, I believe that we have in fact obtained a better bargain in health care — but at a higher cost in human terms than was necessary. Had Canadian governments listened more closely to frontline providers when implementing the necessary changes, we would have achieved the inevitable transformation in a less painful manner. As the new millennium unfolds, the search for value in health services will continue to progress in sophistication. We can hope that policy makers move away from heavy-handed, across-the-board cuts and toward a greater focus on targeted elimination of inappropriate, unnecessary spending. Investment in new kinds of health services for the future is also necessary.

PART II

The Reformation in Health-Care Delivery

5

•

Transforming the Hospital

And what rough beast, Its hour come round at last,
Slouches towards Bethlehem to be born?
— W.B. YEATS, "THE SECOND COMING"

The Calgary General Hospital complex consisted of 850,000 square feet
of hospital buildings on a 12-hectare site in downtown Calgary. The
750,000 residents of the oil capital of Alberta had relied on the General
Hospital for eighty-eight years.

On October 4, 1998, the Calgary General Hospital was completely
destroyed by a series of explosions in a mere twenty-five seconds. This
act of destruction was not the work of terrorists, nor was it an act of God
or a natural-gas rupture. Rather, it was an organized demolition carried
out by the hospital's owner, the Calgary Regional Health Authority. The

hospital was simply no longer needed. A day later, the *Calgary Herald* published a souvenir section to commemorate the historic event. Its headline read, "This is like watching a loved one die."

The Calgary Hospital demolition is a particularly dramatic sign of the transformation that is under way in health services in cities all over the world. Across the industrialized nations we see this same remarkable phenomenon: hospitals are closing, albeit mostly without the aid of dynamite. The most stable and visible symbol of our modern health-care delivery system — the hospital — is radically transforming. Care is being relocated away from the hospital bed, and the time patients spend in hospitals has shortened. Many surgical procedures are now done in a doctor's office, in a day surgery centre without beds, or in the outpatient department of the hospital.

In the United States, the reduction in the number of hospitals is part of the overall consolidation of health care. Major cities often hosted twenty or thirty insurance companies and an equal number of hospitals. Dozens, or even hundreds, of different health plans were available to the employers who paid most insurance premiums directly. Now there are as few as three or four major payers in each region or city — large HMOs (health maintenance organizations) looking for the lowest price and practicing managed care. These changes on the consumer side are leading independent hospitals to similarly consolidate into a few systems serving each major metropolitan area.

As the following table shows, "well-managed" care providers have fewer admissions, much shorter stays, and far fewer total days of use. It is this kind of efficiency that explains the consolidation of acute-care hospitals. "Well-managed" providers are favoured by HMOs for the lower costs that result from their efficiency; more loosely managed hospitals lose patients to these well-managed hospitals, and are likely to set about emulating them to regain their clients.

Comparison of U.S. Managed-Care Providers

	Loosely Managed	Moderately Managed	Well-Managed
Admits per 1,000 Population	83.70	70.80	57.42
Average Length of Stay (Days)	5.38	4.19	3.11
Total Days of Use per 1,000 Population	450.68	296.60	178.45

Source: Milliman and Robertson, 1994.

The Hospital as Cornerstone of the System

For several hundred years, stand-alone hospitals, each with a medical staff, an emergency room, a management team, and a unique set of decisions about which services to provide in-house and which to buy, have been the standard in the developed world. When this model was developed, labour costs were inexpensive; indeed, many early hospitals were staffed by religious women who worked for nothing more than room and board, and the greater glory of God. In Siena, Italy, just outside the town square, is a hospital that has operated since the eleventh century. In many parts of the world, hospitals, often established by religious orders, predate the existence of other institutions, including even the state.

The hospital is, in many ways, a symbol of health care in general. It is one of the most powerful institutions in the modern industrialized world. Standing tall like the great cathedral of the church of health care, it captures the public affection and imagination. The hospital emergency room is what stands between the populace and its fear of the unknown, of illness, of death. We visit emergency rooms at rates far in excess of any objective measure of our need. In 1995, a study in Toronto indicated that, of the 1 million emergency room visits in a year undertaken by the city's 4 million inhabitants, only about 200,000, or 20%, could be justified on the basis of the actual care need. Nevertheless, we persist in our attachment to the hospital as both a cultural and political institution. We judge the performance of health systems by their emergency-room services. As well, a hospital, particularly in a smaller centre, is often an important source of employment; it is usually among a region's major employers.

The pattern of hospital location across North America shows an intriguing continental gradient. The eastern side of the continent has many more hospitals per capita, many of them built in the first 200 to 300 years of development in Canada and the United States. The western side, where population growth came much later, built far fewer inpatient beds. The result is far greater reliance on other (non-inpatient) services in places like California, Oregon, and British Columbia than in New York, Massachusetts, or Ontario. While many East Coast counties and cities consumed, in the mid-1990s, as many as 750 bed days per 1,000 residents per year (meaning that for every thousand people in the local population, there were 750 days of a patient in a hospital bed), the comparable number in parts of western North America was as low as 250 bed days. Are Californians healthier than New Englanders? A little, perhaps. But above all, they are accustomed to drive-in services — fast food, fast gasoline, automated tellers, and health care.

It is estimated that there are 1 million hospital beds in existence in the United States of which only 430,000 are in use. This is the central phenomenon of health-system restructuring: the collapse of inpatient services and their replacement by ambulatory, outpatient, day surgery, and primary-care services. People are no less in need of care, but the location and nature of that care are being transformed.

A Transformation

In this new age, some hospitals are closing, while others are reinventing themselves as part of the networks that are the cornerstone of today's health systems.

The story of U.S. children's hospitals provides an excellent example. Many of these institutions are unique when it comes to tertiary and quarternary services, yet there are a lot of primary and secondary proce- dures that other hospitals can provide more cheaply. These children's hospitals are thus under huge pressure to make one of several choices: to become tertiary; to scale down significantly and just do the things they do uniquely; or to become the hub of a system. Many have chosen the last of these, going into suburban hospitals and proposing, "We'll man- age your pediatrics program."

The Canadian context provides insight into the decline of the hospital. Taking the admission of children to Canadian hospitals as a microcosm of the entire health system is instructive. In 1986/87, some 355,000 Canadian children were admitted to a hospital. A decade later, despite a 10% increase in the child population, only 206,000 children were admitted to Canadian hospitals. The average length of a child's hospital stay also declined by more than half a day, from 4.5 to 3.8 days.

Why this decline? Little has changed in the list of diseases that bring children into the health-care system. Tonsils, adenoids, asthma, and fractures remained the leading causes of hospitalization throughout this period. The key change is the shift from relying primarily on inpa- tient stays to treating the same medical conditions on an outpatient basis. A dramatic increase in day surgery accompanied the decrease in hospital admissions; the setting, not the quantity, of care has changed.

In 1993, the Hospital for Sick Children in Toronto, affectionately known as "Sick Kids'" by locals, opened its beautiful new atrium addi- tion. At a cost of $225 million (CDN), the hospital had added a spectacular, sunlight-filled space to its aging building. But in the ten years that passed between the planning and financing and the new space, much had changed. During the construction process, the hospital had converted many operating rooms in its old section to day surgery sites. After the new wing opened, it became apparent that the inpatient volumes of former times would never return. And yet here stood this magnificent new structure and, more important, an enormously talented group of physicians, nurses, and other professionals with special experience in pediatrics. What was the hospital to do?

Sick Kids' response is typical of the challenge facing many other hospitals: it embarked on a plan to evolve itself into a system, creating a pediatric network serving Toronto's entire population. The plan will probably include closing six or seven of the thirteen pediatric programs in the metropolitan area, consolidating the remaining ones into a network of five pediatric programs, with the Hospital for Sick Children as the hub.

In Toronto, the Hospital for Sick Children has a downtown location. The spread of its pediatrics program to encompass suburban locations like the Mississauga Hospital is being supported by an important computer network; as discussed in Chapter 3, the advances in communication brought about by modern computers have changed the notion of what is possible in terms of administration. In the future, the Mississauga Hospital and others will provide a place for services, but the physicians and the nursing backup will be from the Sick Kids' staff. This approach also helps address the important issue of uneven quality of care in pediatrics. A disbursed program with "quality control" certified by the Hospital for Sick Children is intended to convince parents from across the Toronto region that driving downtown is not their only option for topnotch care from pediatric experts.

Another example of change overtaking expansion plans is Duke University's Medical Center in North Carolina. Its initiatives to reduce inpatient care caused average length of stay at this centre to drop over the course of 5 years from 8.3 to 6.9 days. As a result, Duke scrapped plans for an addition to its 1,124-bed hospital. Instead, the university built an ambulatory surgery centre. Duke's story — the substitution of ambulatory care of inpatient care — is being repeated across the industrialized nations. Empty beds due to shorter lengths of stay are a massive phenomenon across major nations. Once empty beds become numerous, pressures arise to close entire inpatient facilities, or at least cancel plans to expand them.

Growth in the whole health system, but especially in the hospital sector, was fuelled by endlessly increasing funding in the four decades following World War II. When the fiscal squeeze of the 1990s arrived (see Chapter 4), hospitals felt the greatest pressure. Across the industrialized world, hospital funding has been frozen or reduced. Health leaders are finding that they must design health services closer and closer to the populations they serve. Like the square-rigged sailing vessel of centuries past, the stand-alone general hospital is increasingly an anachronism.

Reformers argue we are moving from an antiquated Ptolemaic idea of the health solar system, in which the hospital was the all-powerful core, to a modern Copernican view, in which the rostered patient population is the new sun. The hospital has been reduced from being the sun to being the Pluto of the health solar system. Observers of just a decade or two ago would be astonished indeed to see this powerful institution cast out into the farthest reaches of the health system.

The Evolving Hospital Universe

Current Model

Hospital

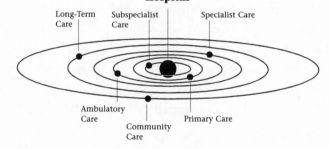

New Model

Rostered Population

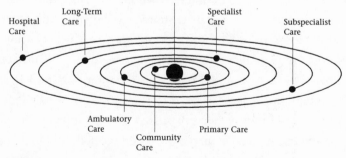

Source: Adapted, with permission, from a presentation given by Roger S. Hunt, President and CEO, Greater Rochester Health System, to the Annual Fellows Dinner of the Canadian College of Health Service Executives, November 4, 1996.

The Four Strong Winds

All four of the forces I described in Part I as reshaping health systems around the globe are felt powerfully in the hospital sector. These strong winds will not abate in the near future, with the exception of some easing of the financial pressure as the economies and fiscal positions of many nations improve.

The situation is complicated, however, by the fact that not all of these forces are driving change in the same direction. For example, financial pressures push hospitals to consolidate in order to achieve efficiencies of scale, while the movement to devolve health services to more local organizations seems to call for smaller institutions. Technological advances allow for wider distribution of information, permitting the sharing of services' decentralized locations, while the current managerial culture of efficiency is creating larger, more centralized health organizations.

The hospital will surely endure as an important institution in each of the industrialized countries. But its role is being reshaped by the forces of new ideas, technology, changing public expectations, and economics. Let us consider each of the forces of change and how it affects the hospital, both as a form of organization and in the larger context of the health system.

Financial constraints tend to cause policy makers — and the public that elects them — to shift their focus from the individual to the system. Looking at hospitals as an industry whole, we find that, while the public expects hospital care to meet standards of quality, these standards do not really exist. In other industries, standards are widely known. For example, when you hear the name "McDonald's," you immediately know what level of food and service that restaurant offers. The same is true for hotels; the name "Holiday Inn" conjures up a fairly accurate image of the type of hotel being discussed. But if you hear the name of a given hospital, it may or may not be connected with an image of the quality of care that this hospital offers. Hospital accreditation — guaranteeing at least a minimum standard — is in some countries still voluntary. Hospitals that receive excellent feedback upon accreditation are of course likely to boast about it, but those that receive poor assessments are not going to tell you about them.

The twenty-first century's hospital sector will be focused on services rather than on beds. Today's hospitals also feature higher acuity levels than yesterday's, meaning that each patient receives more care. Since much simple, low-risk surgery is now done on an outpatient basis, and the increased use of clinics and home care is being encouraged for many kinds of medical problems, the patients who are actually admitted to a hospital bed are much sicker, on average, than they were a decade ago.

The emergence of an organizational form based on hubs and spokes, such as was seen during the development of the airline industry of the 1970s and 1980s, has come to health care. Leading hospitals are extending themselves as the hub of emerging systems. The situation of the Hospital for Sick Children, as recounted above, is not unique: children's hospitals across North America have discovered that, rather than the patients coming to them, they need to take their special expertise and care out to the patients. "Closer to home" has become a theme as payers, be they employers or governments, have sought significant savings in the cost of care.

Hospitals have been labour-intensive beasts, with a tendency to make rather than buy most of the goods and services they have needed, with the exception of drugs and some high-technology services. For many decades, each hospital had its own kitchen, its own laboratory, its own housekeeping staff, and, more recently, sometimes dozens of isolated computer systems that were put together pell-mell as individual physicians and individual departments sought to automate their work.

Today, in regard to computers, the technological revolution has caught up with the modern hospital. As discussed in Chapter 3, increasingly the integration of all information systems in a hospital into one information highway linked to the outside world is driving fundamental changes in such areas as access to information, timeliness of care, and the ability to assess outcomes.

As regards other non-clinical services, the outsourcing revolution has taken hold. Just as other industries have been focusing on their core businesses, the health-care sector, and particularly the hospital, is being forced by financial realities to concentrate on its core competencies. The purpose of hospital health systems may be to treat illness — and perhaps to prevent it — but for several centuries, hospitals have resembled hotels with doctors: their kitchens turned out meals (mostly of dubious culinary merit, albeit nutritious); their laundries processed sheets and soiled garments by the tonne; their labs churned out a multiplicity of test results. This era is coming to an end. Just as the airlines discovered that their core business was flying airplanes and filling them with people, and so contracted out their meal services, so hospitals have turned to outsourcing many of their requirements. Hospital storerooms are disappearing, replaced by the same kind of just-in-time inventory systems that revolutionized the automobile industry.

The parallels between hospitals and auto factories are, in fact, surprisingly strong. Bill Blundell, the retired CEO of General Electric Canada and chair of the Wellesley Hospital Board in Toronto, commented in a 1995 dinner address that what hospitals were going through was very much the same restructuring that had hit the automobile industry. In the old days the famous Rouge Plant of Henry Ford digested tonnes of steel and churned out finished automobiles. Auto makers created cars on huge assembly lines. These days, car plants assemble a multitude of sub-assemblies that have been put together for them by suppliers. Their competency is in assembling the whole car and moving it into the marketplace. Often their financial subsidiaries, which create clever lease and purchase arrangements, are as important to their success as their factories.

This phenomenon of buying from specialist suppliers is seen in virtually every sector of our economy, which is moving toward a more capital-intensive supply chain. The health sector is a latecomer to this transition. Hospitals have remained extraordinarily labour intensive, with, in many cases, 75% to 80% of hospital budgets being paid out in wages. As massive capital investments are made in information systems, and as much of the non-clinical work of hospitals comes to be contracted out, this situation will change. It seems reasonable to expect that labour costs will decline to perhaps 50% to 60% of the overall cost of a health-care system by early in the twenty-first century. Labour costs will remain a higher percentage, perhaps 65% to 70%, of hospital budgets.

This consolidation of non-clinical services is occurring across the industrialized world. From Sydney to Toronto to London, the four winds are blowing hospitals strongly toward consolidation. The pace of change is rapid; after nearly a century of gradual evolution, the hospitals have endured a decade of radical transformation. As the following table underscores, the number of hospital beds per 1,000 people has declined speedily in the past few years, worldwide. In some countries, such as Sweden, the reduction has been truly dramatic.

Overall Changes in Number of Hospital Beds

Country	Hospital Beds per 1,000 People		
	1980	**1993**	**Change**
Netherlands	12.3	11.3	–1.0
Germany	11.5	10.3	–1.2
Finland	15.6	10.0	–5.6
France	11.0	9.4	–1.6
Switzerland	10.0	8.7	–1.3
Italy	9.7	6.9	–2.8
United Kingdom	8.1	5.1	–3.0
Sweden	15.1	7.0	–8.1

Source: OECD Health Data 1998, Paris.

The modern North American hospital was born in Baltimore, Maryland, when a Canadian physician, Dr. William Osler, was hired by the trustees of Johns Hopkins University Hospital. He, in turn, hired a New York hotel manager to serve as his chief administrative officer, and the die was cast. For nearly a century thereafter, hospitals would be conceived of as hotels with doctors and nurses. Like hotels, they measured their performance by occupancy rates and their importance by numbers of beds.

In today's reconfigured hospital, outsourcing means that many non-clinical functions take place away from the physical site of the hospital. Central laundries return clean uniforms by the truckload. Centralized kitchens deliver prepared meals to be reheated. Larger, more centralized laboratories send back test results over the Internet. The hospital, like the automobile factory before it, has moved from building patient care from scratch to assembling its parts, manufactured elsewhere. The evolving hospital is in need of expertise to manage its new relationships with partners and suppliers.

The 1990s have ushered in the most rapid and profound change to the hospital since Dr. Osler. The powerful forces of new organizational forms, automation, and new medical technologies that favour ambulatory care, all driven by a relentless cost-cutting and efficiency drive, have combined to reshape the hospital sector dramatically and rapidly. For the first time in a century, a decade will end with fewer hospitals in each of the industrialized countries than there were at its beginning. Hospital closures, a hitherto rare phenomenon, have become commonplace — if still controversial. The remaining hospitals are reshaping their roles, becoming managers of health services rather than managers of beds. Services, not beds, are the measure of the performance of a modern hospital.

If the old-style hospital was like a hotel in organization, it was like a grand department store in terms of the range of goods and services on offer. All services were available. The emerging hospital of the new millennium owes more of its heritage to the shopping mall: a collection of boutique services in special niches. Typically, in major cities, large general hospitals are giving way to more specialized institutions that are likely to refer patients elsewhere for specific services they themselves do not offer. This shift in the role of the hospital needs to be accompanied by an increase in ambulatory and home services — a profound and seemingly permanent shift driven by the progress of modern medications, the advances of minimally invasive surgery, and the advent of more robust home health services. The expansion of non-hospital services often lags behind the consolidation of hospitals. This problem is evident in overcrowded emergency rooms, patient dissatisfaction, and newspaper headlines screaming "Health-care Crisis!"

The Canadian Experience

At the beginning of the 1990s, Canada had approximately 900 hospitals. Each one had its own governing body, management team, and physical facility. From the late 1950s on, the funding for hospitals came largely from provincial governments, which provided global budgets for hospitals. This system of hospital financing continued for thirty years with little change. Only in the early 1990s did the rate of increase in spending decline and the method of payment begin to shift, from global budgets that rewarded hospitals for simply existing to systems that rewarded efficiency and volume.

In Canada, the provincial governments play the dominant role in funding health-care services. Each province has initiated its own health-restructuring initiatives during the 1990s, embarking on a process of consolidation and regionalization of the Canadian hospital and health systems. There have been differences in the approach taken by each of the ten provinces, but the general pattern has been the same: a move toward fewer governing bodies and larger, more geographically based delivery organizations. The form these changes have taken has ranged from multi-site hospital corporations to much broader health services–delivery organizations. The creation of new, regional health authorities represents a devolution of authority down from the provincial level, but also a consolidation of authority up from dozens of hospital boards and other health organizations, such as, in many cases, nursing homes. Multi-site hospital organizations were rare phenomena in Canada a decade ago, but are rapidly becoming the dominant organizational form.

The shortening of hospital stays in Canada led first to hospital bed closures, then, more recently, to the closure of entire hospitals. The two dominant criteria in the decisions regarding which hospitals to eliminate have been the age and condition of physical facilities and their proximity to centres of population growth. Older, inner-city hospitals have been most vulnerable to closure, along with small-town hospitals in areas of where the population is declining.

Canadian hospital expenditures have, in keeping with total health expenditures, been growing more slowly in recent years, and in some years have actually shown an absolute decline: from 1994 to 1997, total hospital spending in current dollars went down by a little more than 1% per year. Even more tellingly, the *share* of total Canadian health expenditures accounted for by hospitals has also declined. In 1976, they represented 45.4% of total Canadian health spending. By 1995, the share was only 35.5%. An increase in spending on drugs is the most important factor responsible for this shift (see Chapter 8 for more on drug therapy and associated spending).

The U.S. Experience

In 1995, the United States had 1.2 million hospital beds available, but only 639,000 were occupied. The occupancy level by 1999 had further fallen to about 440,000. The winds of change blowing through health systems are pushing many nations in the same direction: in the United States, too, stand-alone, acute-care hospitals are consolidating into larger groupings and agglomerations. And, be they called integrated health systems or networks or regions, these new entities are larger and more complex than the old ones.

I once had the privilege of sharing a podium with Dr. John Hassells, the president emeritus of Johns Hopkins Medical Center, which is frequently ranked as the leading medical centre in the United States. Dr. Hassells explained that one of his very good friends was the manager of a chain of department store, The May Department Stores, while he viewed Johns Hopkins as the last great department store, albeit medical, in downtown Baltimore. He commented that every time Johns Hopkins was convinced to move some service to the suburban clinic setting on the basis that it would direct business back to the downtown hospital, this never happened. The business stayed out there in the suburban clinic setting. His view was that the era of great department stores in health care — the large downtown hospital — was ending, just as the era of great department stores in retailing has given way to an uneasy coexistence of suburban malls, which offer convenience and speed, and downtown department stores, which offer character and depth of merchandise. So, too, in the health-care sector, one expects that many frequently used primary and secondary services will migrate closer to where our populations now live, while tertiary and quaternary (specialized) services remain in more central institutions.

Whither the Teaching Hospital?

The department-store hospital's days may be numbered, but academic medical centres like Johns Hopkins have displayed an extraordinary ability to adapt. These are truly, in American business analyst Peter Senge's language, learning organizations, and they will continue to have an important role as innovators, teaching centres, and, through example, leaders in patient care. In fact, Senge, in a Vancouver presentation, identified academic medical centres as the most complex organizations created on Earth. The combination of scientists and clinicians and the triple mandate of teaching, research, and practice all contribute to this complexity. Increasingly, the research and teaching roles are under financial pressure from cost containment in care delivery.

What extra financial rewards society is willing to confer to keep these academic medical centres current is not yet clear. In the United Kingdom, the 1993 Sifter Proposal for funding of health care provides for a 20% to 30% larger budget for teaching centres. Historically, in the United States, a similar bonus has been available. However, the business-oriented U.S. payer community is increasingly less sensitive to academic and research arguments. Their view is that their mandate is to buy services at the most efficient price point, and if these can all be obtained more affordably and at similar quality from suburban, non-teaching medical centres, then they will take that option.

Around the world, those who administer academic medical centres, as well as the physicians who work within them, are trying to understand their fall from the pedestal, and seeking the best ways to manage the transition. Their task will be a challenging one in a cost-driven, restructured health-care delivery world.

The Funding Dilemma

In part, the emergence of larger organizations to deliver health services comes from the intensification of capital investment required in the sector. Traditionally, hospitals have spent a very small percentage — perhaps 1% to 2% of their budgets — on information technology. Capital funding for hospitals in many nations is extremely limited and has been driven by charitable fundraising activities for the most part. This private model of funding was up to the task of building a new wing once a decade, or a new hospital once in a generation, but is clearly insufficient for meeting the significant, ongoing capital requirements of today's complex health organizations. The requirement for up-to-date, well-managed, and, frankly, expensive information systems is one of the most significant results of the emergence of larger organizations. It is also a driving cause of further amalgamation in the health sector. Larger organizations can more readily raise the needed capital.

Now What?

Health systems cling to the status quo with extraordinary tenacity. However, the four strong winds of change are moving society to a new place in health care despite all resistance. The clear response to fragmented, uncoordinated, health-care systems and a lack of measurable outcomes is a move toward larger, integrated health organizations, and a change in the very meaning of the term "hospital" is a necessary part of this move.

The hospitals of North America are not simply being closed or merged; they are also being reengineered, following, for the most part, the same principles that swept industrial reengineering a decade or two ago. The traditional hospital was like a large, not very efficient factory. Just as the manufacturing sector, driven by competitive pressures, restructured its work processes, changing its whole approach to making products, so too does the hospital of today seek efficiencies wherever it can, through, for example:

◇ supply-chain management;
◇ consolidation of back-office functions;
◇ redesign of care delivery; and
◇ reorganization of work.

So far, some of the factory-inspired techniques for increasing efficiency have worked extremely well in the hospital sector. The consolidation and outsourcing of support functions such as food services and laboratory testing have achieved significant savings.

More detailed examples of integrated health-care delivery systems, including their effect in hospitals, are discussed in Chapters 11 through 14, where I try to identify some key ideas and lessons relating to each of these examples. We need to learn from the pioneers — both their triumphs and their failures can provide valuable teachings. The views of critics from outside the system are also important, reminding us to examine the gap between expectations and achievements.

Many important questions relating to the hospital sector remain unanswered. What is the most efficient scale for a hospital facility? How many people can be looked after effectively by a single hospital system? What is the role of a hospital in improving the general health of a population? Only time and trials will tell.

I can, however, based on recent trends, make a few predictions about how the place and function of acute-care hospitals are likely to evolve in the next decade:

◇ fewer hospitals subsumed into more complex, multi-site health-delivery organizations in North America — perhaps 2,000 to 3,000 systems in North America instead of the 9,000 individual hospitals of today;
◇ higher acuity (sicker patients) in inpatient settings;
◇ rapid growth in ambulatory/day procedures and facilities;
◇ high levels of information technology change, including increased links among providers;
◇ greater availability of consumer-useable information regarding quality and outcomes, leading to more "shopping" among providers;

◇ more capital investment;
◇ less reliance on unskilled labour;
◇ more narrowly focused specialty hospitals in some niche services; and
◇ the greater involvement of hospitals in defining their role within a continuum of care or disease-state management programs.

Hospitals are unlikely to easily relinquish the affection of the public as a critically important element of the health-care system. But they will have to make room for the expanding role of other parts of the system, resigning themselves to a position that looks less like galactic domination and more like *primus inter pares*.

6

•

New Physicians' Organizations: Is Dr. Kildare Dead?

Nine of ten doctors complained about health organizations reject-ing services for their patients.
— KAISER FAMILY FOUNDATION SURVEY (1999)

The last decade of the twentieth century saw an unusually savage conflict between the forces of change and the entrenched power of the medical profession. This conflict was felt worldwide, but took different forms in different nations. The result is that many doctors have ended up feeling set upon, unloved, besieged in their own countries.

Have we turned against our doctors? I don't believe we have. But our society's relationship with our doctors is undergoing a fundamental change. This transformation, brought about by the same four winds of change that are reinventing other aspects of our health systems, is very difficult for medical practitioners, particularly those with many years in practice, to understand. It is even more difficult for them to accept.

The term "primary-care reform" has become a mantra in health policy circles. Many different meanings can be attributed to these three words — and some of these differing interpretations represent a direct challenge to doctors' power.

Down from the Pedestal

British scholar Rudolf Klein offers a profound insight into the nature of the transformation of the relationship between doctors and society. Historically, doctors, Klein explains, have enjoyed a relationship with society based on status. They were not questioned. They were largely accountable to other doctors, but not to the society in general. Status — high status — characterized all aspects of the doctor-society relationship, including pay, conduct, and power structure.

All that is changing rapidly — too rapidly for many doctors to accept the new ways. Klein argues that the new relationship between doctors and society is a "contract" relationship. This term does not refer to a literal contract, although in some American health maintenance organizations (HMOs) actual physician contracts are, in fact, common, and they are also found in the United Kingdom. But what Klein means is that doctors have seen their relationships with the communities they serve made more explicit. As the status of doctors has declined, as they have come down off their pedestals in the minds of the general public, a great questioning, heretofore unthinkable, has begun. How should doctors behave? How should they be paid? How should their competency be ensured? How should their professional judgment be assessed? The answers to questions such as these form the "contract" relationship at the heart of the new doctor-society bargain.

It has been a bruising time for a profession long used to a status afforded few others. Medicine has remained almost the last of the medieval guilds: self-regulating and powerful. Yet even this guild, after centuries of dominating health care, is succumbing to the powerful winds of change. Debates have sprung up around the world about doctors' place, shaped by the history of each country's particular relationship between physicians and the rest of the health-care system.

British reforms focused on changing the role of the general practitioner. The power of the specialist was seen as a major barrier to improved efficiency and better responsiveness to consumer pressures; the balance of power has now shifted to favour family doctors, with beneficial results in the delivery of health-care services.

In the United States, the forces of the market and the power of major corporations as exercised through HMOs have challenged physicians' traditional power. The new, cost-conscious insurers have focused on the cost and appropriateness of care. The insistence of many HMOs and insurers on managing physicians closely, requiring prior approval before medical procedures can go ahead, has provoked a backlash among both physicians and patients.

American legislators have responded to this backlash, passing "patient bills of rights." In his 2000 State of the Union Address, President Clinton promised a National Patient Bill of Rights. The next step forward in this battle is the courtroom, where legislators' authority will be tested against that of the physicians they would control.

In Canada, the debate has been more muted. Consumers have difficulty deciding how to allocate blame between governments and doctors for the troubles they see in their health-care system. But any smugness Canadians might have enjoyed regarding the stability of their system relative to the U.S. one evaporated in the 1990s' stressful and controversial restructuring of hospitals. Canadian provincial governments have also squeezed physicians' incomes without changing the nature of the payment system for them, a move that has prompted its own fair share of controversy and public debate.

The Direction of the Winds

The winds of health-care change have brought us, here in Canada, new forms of physician organizations, new ways of paying for doctors' services, and an increased emphasis on primary care. As the delivery of health care becomes more tightly managed, patient care is shifting away from acute-care hospitals and into the community and family setting. But unless the primary-care system is ready for this shift, with nurses, doctors, pharmacists, and others available in community and home settings, patients will return to the hospitals, taxing the capacity of emergency rooms and, along the way, damaging public confidence in health-care services as the nightly news features story after story of over-crowding. In the wake of a decade of hospital restructuring, attention has now turned to the urgent need for a reformed approach to primary care. Here as in other nations, efforts to invest more health-care dollars in home and community care are under way.

New Forms of Physicians' Organizations

Why are the upheavals in the system creating new forms of physicians' organizations?

First, where the money squeeze is sharpest, the impetus to seek effi-ciencies is strong (see Chapter 4). The most obvious efficiencies are ones of scale; in the case of physicians' organizations, this suggests a move toward group practice. Efficiencies also require more effective practice management — something that can be achieved through more formal organization. New public expectations (such as speed, quality, and appro-priateness, as discussed in Chapter 2) are also compelling larger-scale physician organizations, since patient expectations of fast, quality service on a twenty-four-hour, seven-days-a-week basis cannot be met by solo physicians. Nor can physicians' own growing information needs; the in-formation technology systems required to handle today's huge quantities of medical data require significant capital investment and maintenance funds, which a larger group of physicians can shoulder more easily.

The United Kingdom led primary-care reform in the 1940s and 1950s, when it introduced to the National Health Service significant incentives for physicians operating in practice groups. In most other countries, however, physician practice has, until recently, continued to consist largely of solo practices, leaving practitioners without the benefits of substituting other providers and without the ability to acquire leading information technology.

So-called physician-hospital links connect a capitated physician practice (one in which physicians are paid an amount for each enrolled patient per month, rather than for each service rendered) with a hospital system, creating vertical integration of acute and primary care. Cost savings are achieved by looking after patients more effectively in their own homes or communities under the supervision of other health-care workers, enabling patients to stay out of costly acute-care hospitals. In essence, these linkages provide a more robust form of primary care connected to a leaner hospital system.

The emergence of new forms of physician organizations has not been as universal a phenomenon as the consolidation of hospitals into larger health services organizations. But there is some significant movement in many countries toward a capitated-funding model for an enrolled population. The chart on pages 80–81 shows some of these initiatives.

In 1995, the Canadian government released the Kilshaw Report, which advocated moving primary care in Canada away from solo practices and the fee-for-service model, and toward formal primary-care organizations in which groups of physicians take responsibility for the care of certain populations. The immediate reaction of medical associations was negative, but one expects that, as with many other key innovations, these changes, once implemented, will be embraced by the physician community as the new status quo, and hence defended against all future change.

The Canadian Experience: A Few Tentative Steps

Beyond a handful of pilot projects, Canada has seen little actual change to its fee-for-service, physician-based primary care until recently. It has lagged behind other nations in organizing a more robust, multi-professional, primary-care service. Canadians generally thought themselves as well served by a primary-care approach based almost entirely on family

Some Capitation-Funding Initiatives

Jurisdiction	Program	Services Included	Parallel Funding Methods
Finland	Population Responsibility System	• primary care services • prevention	salary fee-for-service
Netherlands	(i) Social Health Insurance (Sickness Funds)	• primary care services • secondary care services • acute hospital care • pharmaceuticals	fee-for-service
	(ii) Primary Care Capitation (for beneficiaries of insurance from Sickness Funds)	• primary care services • GPs determine the basic package of services to provide	none
New Zealand	(i) Budget-Holding Contracts	• laboratory services • subsidized pharmaceuticals	none
	(ii) Capitation Funding for General Practitioners	• primary care services	fee-for-service
Norway	Primary-Care Pilot Projects	• primary care services • a defined set of preventive services	blended funding of fee-for-service and salary

United Kingdom	(i) General Practitioner Capitation	• primary-care services • health-promotion and disease-prevention services	none

	(ii) General Practitioner Fundholding	Standard fundholding:
		• hospital inpatient care (defined list of services)
		• outpatient visits
		• diagnostic services
		• drugs
		• practice staff management allowance
		Total fundholding:
		• the above set of services plus:
		  – community-based care
		  – other inpatient care
			none

United States	Medicare Program	• primary-care services • specialist physicians' services • diagnostic services • hospital inpatient care	fee-for-service

Note: There are varying arrangements for seeing patients in the private sector, which are not reflected in these tables.

Source: Canadian Health Services Research Foundation, *Policy Synthesis: Policy Considerations in Implementing Capitation for Integrated Health Systems*, March 1999.

doctors. But today the shifting gender mix in family practice — there are many more women — and the increasing reluctance of family doctors to work evenings and weekends is forcing change. Small communities across Canada have faced physician shortages for years, and the situation worsened significantly in the late 1990s.

In October 1999, a small tender ad was placed by the Ontario Ministry of Health. It sought eighty-six nurse practitioners to "provide primary health care across the province, especially in designated underserviced areas and northern communities." There are also a number of physician-led primary-care pilot projects under way in Ontario. These projects seek to change physician practice by financially rewarding preventive care. Other provinces are also moving slowly into this area. The early part of the new century will witness difficult negotiations between the Canadian medical profession and the various provincial governments as we develop a reformed approach to the community-based practice of medicine.

The U.S. Experience: Physicians, Inc.

Fed up wrestling with the nine expanding health maintenance organizations operating in Cincinnati, Ohio, internist Dr. Donald Saelinger and twenty-nine associates sold their practices. His reasoning was simple: "If you are a small doctor group, you will not be able to make a living." Already in Cincinnati, internists, family practitioners, and pediatricians have seen their incomes drop 10% from two years ago. Specialists' fees have fallen by as much as 50%. The result seems to be a further step toward capitation.

One example of a new American response to the upheavals in how medicine in that country is managed and paid for is PhyCor, Inc., which bills itself as "the physician's corporation." It is a creation of the capital markets that have begun financing the growth of physician management businesses. Headquartered in Nashville, Tennessee, PhyCor is a medical network management company that operates multi-specialty medical clinics and independent practice associations (IPAs) and provides health-care decision-support services to consumers. As of 1998, it operated 56 clinics with more than 3,500 physicians in 27 states and managed IPAs with approximately 22,900 physicians in 35 markets, holding responsibility for the health care of more than 1.5 million people.

PhyCor sets out its approach and history as follows:

> Our basic underlying concept . . . remains the foundation of the reform movement. It is the decisions of physicians that drive the cost and quality of health care. Physicians only receive around 20% of health-care expenditures as they manage the diagnosis, treatment, and care of their patients. It is acceptable that physician performance will determine the value in competitive networks as we move from treating illness to managing care and ultimately the health of a population. PhyCor provides a vehicle for physicians to maximize their performance and thus the competitiveness of their evolving networks. . . . The organization that has the most competitive structure is the primary-care balanced, multi-specialty physician group. Today, PhyCor is nationally recognized as the pioneer and leader in what is now identified as the physician practice management sector of the health-care system.

PhyCor has become national in scope and ambition. It has affiliated itself with physician groups in every quadrant of the United States, operating in all types of markets: rural, regional, and urban. The group sizes vary from dozens to hundreds of physicians. PhyCor is also one of the nation's largest operators of IPAs as a complement to its core physician-group business.

PhyCor operates medical clinics in conjunction with physician group practices. The physicians practise medicine while PhyCor provides business skills and financial resources. PhyCor invests in the clinic and receives certain assets in exchange, thus becoming the "corporate partner" of the medical group. This transaction allows the medical group to make liquid a portion of their equity, which produces retained earnings.

The medical group retains control over the direction of the medical practice. A joint policy board, composed of representatives from PhyCor, local clinic management, and the physician group, establishes policies and oversees the operation of the clinic. A new operating structure is thereby created.

Physicians all over the country face the same issues and, more than ever, need the capital, management, and organizational resources of corporations like PhyCor. Hospitals have historically seen physician-management companies as competitors, increasingly viewing corporations such as PhyCor as partners in physician strategies that can contribute strengths to their financial position and to care management.

PhyCor has recently expanded to form a health-information company, called CareWise, which provides medical-decision support services. It offers a wide range of health information and call centres where individuals can talk with nurses about health situations. PhyCor hopes to link physicians and consumers through this organization, which is based on rapidly advancing information and telecommunication technology, including the Internet. This company is intended to become an integrated part of PhyCor, just as the IPA business has.

PhyCor is an example of the emerging corporate model of physician practice management in the United States.

The British Experience: GP Fundholding

Clearly the most radical reform undertaken by the National Health Service since its inception has been GP fundholding. The notion is simple: general practitioners act as informed purchasers of care for their patients. They are given budgets to purchase prescription drugs as well as hospital services, such as laboratory tests, outpatient ambulatory care, and certain elective operations.

The impressive pace at which GP fundholding expanded in the United Kingdom is worthy of note — from less than 10% in 1991/92 to nearly 60% of general practitioners a mere six years later.

The Labour government of Tony Blair came to power promising to abolish GP fundholding, but ended up retaining much of the reform. A June 1999 editorial in the *Evening Standard* explains:

The Rise of GP Fundholding

Year	General Practitioner Coverage %
1991–92	7
1992–93	13
1993–94	25
1994–95	35
1995–96	41
1996–97	53
1997–98	59

Source: David Knowles, "Policy Developments: British Healthcare Reform Through Internal Markets and Beyond." Presentation to the OHA convention, Toronto, November 4, 1997.

Many commentators greeted the Labour Government's New National Health Service White Paper as evolutionary. GP fundholding was to be abolished but many elements of the internal market have, in practice, been retained. Primary Care Groups, the vehicles for delivering much new health policy, represent an amalgam of previous models.* They are charged with three objectives:

— improving the health of the population and addressing health inequalities;
— developing primary and community health services; and
— commissioning appropriate hospital services.

The new Primary Care Programme is heavily focused on the development of Primary Care Groups in London with projects linking across all other programmes. Building on the national evaluation of Purchasing Pilots, the PCP is being commissioned by the National Health Service executive to undertake elements of

---

* Primary Care Groups make up a new health service organization that provides medical, nursing, and social services to elderly and long-term disability patients in a community, not a hospital, setting.

a national programme of evaluation. Early mapping work has underlined the extent of the organizational challenge in developing these new bodies.

Other creations of the old regime have been continued and adapted by the Blair government in areas of physician management and primary care:

◇ personal medical services pilots, which were permitted by the 1997 Primary Care Act, and may be critical in the formation of Primary Care Trusts;
◇ primary-care trusts, to manage primary care under a government board;
◇ nurse-led teams providing primary care; and
◇ an increase in those served by general practitioners and others working outside the national contract under innovative physician arrangements — nearly 20% of London's population by the year 2001.

One fundamental obstacle to health-service integration in the United Kingdom has been the tripartite division of care into hospital, community, and family practitioner services, combined with the independent contractor status of general practitioners. The move to unify budgets that embrace hospital and community health-care services, cash-limited general medical services, and prescribing budgets therefore represents an important advance.

The United Kingdom is once again in a time of further organizational upheaval, featuring some of the same problems as those that accompanied the reforms of the early 1990s: a preoccupation with structures, a miring in organizational process, and a sense that Primary Care Group board members are "learning by doing." As the role of health professionals in primary care is changing, so are managerial roles. There is a danger of putting too much emphasis on the boat and not enough on the winds.

One of the leading foundations for research, teaching, and advocacy in health in the United Kingdom is the King's Fund. Created a hundred years ago, its full title is King Edward's Hospital Fund for London. The

King's Fund is undertaking a survey of Londoners' views on primary care in collaboration with the *Evening Standard* to determine the patient impact of proposed reforms. In anticipation of the results, an *Evening Standard* editorial points out the following:

> It is tempting to conclude, when only a tiny proportion of the population have even heard of Primary Care Groups, that much of the organizational froth and bother will pass the public by. It is here that the government's reforms pass the real tests of revolutionary intent. The expansion of National Health Service Direct as the first point of contact for people seeking medical care will transform the public's perceptions of the service. Taken together, these changes will alter primary care professionals' working lives in ways yet unforeseen.

Conclusions

What can we conclude from the disparate experiences of three nations regarding the organization of physicians?

First, that change is difficult when it involves a profession with as much history, status, and power as medicine. The Canadian experience shows that physicians can successfully block change in politically managed health systems.

Second, the direction of change is clear: the developed world is moving toward larger physician groups that are more formally linked to the rest of the health system. So, too, is there a pushing down of risk from the payer level to the physician-group level.

Finally, an increased emphasis on primary care — both physician-led and nurse-led — is emerging. In the face of consolidation in the acute-care hospital sector, leading to shorter stays and fewer beds, the cry for a more robust primary-care system is echoing demands from both patients and their families and also from beleaguered emergency departments, which is the refuge of the worried patient in the absence of quality, convenient primary-care options in the community.

7

•

Nursing in the New Order

Nursing is managing.

— PROFESSOR HENRY MINTZBERG

The 1990s have proven an extremely tough decade for the nursing profession. Across the industrialized countries, heated debate rages about the current state and future prospects of this time-honoured profession. These debates are not only within the nursing community; they also spill out to engage and, sometimes, to alarm the public. Many industrialized countries are swinging rapidly from having a nursing surplus to being in a severe nursing shortage.

Some argue that nursing is being de-skilled, citing as evidence the massive reduction of hospital-based nurses and their replacement by less-skilled professionals. Within the ranks of nursing, critics note a shift from highly skilled registered nurses to less-skilled licensed practical

nurses. Others point to the professionalization of nursing, the requirement that anyone entering nursing today have a bachelor's degree,
and the rapid growth in specialized areas of nursing. Still others
note the shift of nursing from the hospital to the community, and
from a charitable activity to one increasingly run by for-profit corporate
organizations.

What is going on with nursing? Is the spirit of Florence Nightingale
dead? Have the values underlying nursing given away to unionism in
a corporate market setting? The answer is that all of the above are likely
true. A nurse is no longer just a nurse; there are many varieties of nurses
and many different sets of circumstances.

It is clear that in some circumstances, nurses' work *has* been devalued.
Nurses have been moved out of the skilled labour force and their
work taken over in part by those without nursing training or skills. It
is equally true that, in other circumstances, nurses were in fact doing
a great deal of work that was not really nursing work. Moving that work
to others has freed up nurses to do their real jobs better.

Scientific Support for Skilled Nurses

Professor Henry Mintzberg, the leading expert on organizational theory
quoted in the chapter opening, is also of the view that nurses should
be empowered in the hospital. He suggests that this change should come
by "disempowering" physicians. Nurses, Mintzberg argues, manage care
well and should have more responsibility in the hospital setting.

As the evidence-based revolution grips the health system, groups such
as nurses are being asked to back up claims of the importance of their
role with more than history. Dr. Linda Aiken, who runs the Center for
Health Services and Policy Research at the University of Pennsylvania,
has risen to this challenge. Dr. Aiken has been working to link quality of
nursing to patient outcomes through research. The essence of her findings to date is that there is a direct connection between patients'
outcomes and the skill level of the nursing staff involved in those
patients' care. This finding is not surprising to anyone in the health

system, but Dr. Aiken's work documents the connection scientifically. This study is being replicated across a number of industrialized countries; more results are expected before too long.

Of course, the emergence of a formal body of statistical data supporting the link between patient outcomes and quality of nursing care will not end the debate. But it will certainly energize nurses in pressing their demands — and perhaps make patients and voters their allies.

The "Where" of Care

The venue for nursing work is also changing. Historically, nurses worked on the battlefield and the home, but eventually they came to be most identified with the hospital. Thus, as the hospital has been transformed and downsized (see Chapter 5), much of the nursing work formerly performed there has been eliminated. New technologies, shorter stays, and fewer hospital beds have all reduced many of the traditional roles of hospital nurses.

But these changes have not eliminated the importance of nursing so much as shifted it. Reforms in many countries have failed to take into account the need for nursing care — and the dollars to fund it — to follow patients as they are moved out of the hospital setting and into the community and their homes. Only when the health systems in these nations reinvest in more broadly defined health-care delivery are the concerns of nurses — and of their patients — likely to be put to rest.

The 1990s were a decade of massive upheaval for nursing. Tens of thousands of North American nurses were displaced from their jobs in the hospital sector. As we enter the twenty-first century, it is evident to many in health care that a new role is being created for nurses. More accurately, some aspects of an old role are being rediscovered, such as home health care, patient education, and serving as a compassionate adviser to patients.

In this new role, a lot of nursing activity can take place in a call centre and on the Internet. Nurse telephone services — with names like Call a Nurse, Ask a Nurse, and Nurse on Call — have become an important dimension of primary care in a number of countries, including Canada. As telehealth continues to expand, so will telenursing.

The forms that this nursing care has taken vary by country. In the United Kingdom, The Caring Network, operated by the British company Tunstall, contracts with housing authorities to provide nursing care over the telephone to residents of council flats — part of an effort to keep the elderly in their homes longer. In the United States, Access Health puts nurses on telephone lines to assist with triage for members of HMOs who might otherwise appear at the emergency rooms of local hospitals. The cost per call of approximately $10 (U.S.) is readily borne by HMOs, as an emergency-room visit can cost ten times as much. Patients can now receive over the phone a great deal of the information that they could have obtained in the past only by visiting a health professional in person.

Nurse Practitioners

The restructuring of primary care has also seen a resurgence in the use of nurse practitioners. These professionals are increasingly sought after in health systems to undertake tasks such as diagnosing certain patients, prescribing drugs, and undertaking some kinds of treatment. In Ontario, these practitioners have been given a specific legal framework under which they can provide such services — all of which trained nurses have demonstrated great success in providing. Nurse practitioners are not junior doctors; the work they undertake is nursing work, with an expanded scope based upon an expanded skill base.

Anne Marie Rafferty, a passionate nursing advocate, runs the Centre for Policy in Nursing Research at the London School of Hygiene and Tropical Medicine in the U.K. Her views, noted in several published works, focus on the history and role of nursing. One of her conclusions is that the struggle of nurses for their place in health-care systems is essentially a political struggle for power against the more powerful physicians' guilds.

A 1996 monograph by Dr. Judith Shamian and Dr. Beverly Chambers of the WHO Collaborating Centre and the University of Toronto included the following points of evidence:

◇ The first major review of the role and value of the nurse practitioner, carried out by the U.S. Congress Office of Technology Assessment in 1986, concluded that the care provided by nurse practitioners is equivalent in quality to that provided by physicians.

◇ The same study found that, in areas of communication and preventive care, nurse practitioners were more adept than physicians.

◇ A 1987 review of 248 papers on the effectiveness of nurse practitioners in such areas as diagnosing problems, providing patient teaching, counselling and follow-up care, collaborating with other health professionals, seeking consultations, making referrals, performing physical exams, taking histories, ordering diagnostic exams, and prescribing treatments, as well as achieving a variety of positive patient-related outcomes, such as increased health knowledge, compliance, health maintenance, follow-up return, accessibility of care, decreased incidence and length of hospitalization and number of inpatient days, and satisfaction of both patient and employer, found:

— that patients are satisfied with the care provided by nurse practitioners;

— that the interpersonal skills of nurse practitioners are better than those of physicians;

— that the technical quality of nurse practitioner services is equivalent to that of physician services;

— that nurse practitioner outcomes are equivalent or superior to physician patient outcomes; and

— that nurse practitioners facilitate continuity of patient care, improved access to care in rural and other settings, and the provision of care to underserved populations (Crosby, Ventura, and Feldman, 1987).

◇ A more recent meta-analysis of the role and impact of nurse practitioners confirms these conclusions (Brown & Grimes, 1993). Outcomes of this meta-analysis reveal that nurse practitioners provided more health promotion than physicians, scored higher on quality-of-care measures than physicians, prescribed drugs at equivalent rates, ordered more laboratory tests (although the average cost for these was lower), were more successful at resolving pathological conditions and improving the functional status of their patients, achieved higher scores than physicians on patient satisfaction and compliance, and spent on average 50% more time with their patients — all at an average cost per visit of only about two-thirds that of a physician.

Is it any wonder that many nations are seeking a greater role for nurse practitioners in primary care?

Conclusions

Despite these and many other studies offering evidence that nurses do a better job in many aspects of primary care, industrialized nations continue to give physicians leadership in or sole responsibility for primary care, almost without exception. Why, at a time when one of the great health-care cries is for more evidence-based practice, does this gap between evidence and practice persist? The power of the medical profession has been reduced a little, in relation to nursing, but no fundamental rebalancing has occurred in most nations.

If a such a shift did occur, what would we do with all these physicians? The rostering of patients has already led to significant unemployment among physicians in parts of Europe. In health policy, simply having solid evidence on the side of an idea is not a guarantee of change.

Nurses now play a prominent role in providing health information over the telephone — just as they have for centuries at the bedside. As telehealth expands, the role of nurses as advisers and as triage agents will continue to grow.

Suzanne Gordon, in the preface to her excellent 1998 book *Life Support: Three Nurses on the Front Lines*, comments that "[n]ursing may be the oldest art, but in the contemporary world, it is also one of the most invisible. One of the most invisible arts, sciences, and certainly one of the most invisible parts of our health-care system." Yet as nursing moves from hospital to community and home, and as it struggles to find a new financial base, it is becoming more visible. If policy makers can be encouraged to include a true measure of the contribution of nursing in the evidence-based revolution, this movement will help nurses find their fullest role in reforming the delivery of care.

Claire Fagin, dean emeritus of the University of Pennsylvania School of Nursing, describes the nursing mission thus in her introduction to Suzanne Gordon's book: "Throughout its history, the profession of nursing has woven all that nurses know and do into an integrated and seamless tapestry of care." This tapestry is somewhat torn and twisted these days in the upheaval of the hospital sector; it seems that only as damage is done are health-policy makers and managers realizing the essential, integrating quality of nursing. As the quest for truly integrated patient care gains momentum, I trust that a revitalized central role for nursing will develop.

8

•

New Drugs, New Challenges

The very strength of the upcycle in the drug industry over the past five years appears to be sowing the seeds for a new round of cost containment. . . .

— Merrill Lynch, *Global Pharmaceuticals Research Report* (December 1999)

Drugs were the main event in twentieth-century medicine. Medication emerged as the most potent tool we have to prevent and treat illness — the share of health spending devoted to drugs worldwide has grown steadily. In terms of sheer quantity, the world's annual market for pharmaceuticals is astronomical — estimated at more than $300 billion (U.S.) in 1998, and growing at about 7% to 8% a year. This growth is driven by the introduction of new products; the pharmaceutical industry invests an estimated $40 billion a year in research and development. Much of the progress made in health services in the twentieth century came from a few new classes of drugs, such as antibiotics and insulin. Whole classes of life-threatening diseases were vanquished in less than a generation by drugs and vaccines.

Spiralling Costs

The cost of developing a new drug has escalated as the time it takes to get it safely and legally to market has lengthened. The Pharmaceutical Research and Manufacturers Association has estimated that over the course of a little over twenty years, the average time to develop a drug increased by over 30%, from eleven years to over fifteen years. In the United States, the average number of Phase I to Phase III clinical trials per new drug application has doubled from the 1970s to the 1990s. (Drugs are tested first on animals and then, in three phases, on humans for safety and then efficacy.) And as the number of trials increased over this period, so did the number of patients in the clinical development program, by about 2,000 patients per new drug application. As a result, the total cost of developing a new drug increased astronomically — from an average of about $54 million (U.S.) in 1976 to $360 million in 1990, a rise of about 500%.

Cost Containment

It is not surprising, therefore, that costs to the consumer have gone up, too. In fact, drug costs have risen faster than all other aspects of health care. The chief actuary of Empire Blue Cross/Blue Shield in New York recently noted this shift. In 1996, inpatient hospital care accounted for 22% of total health-plan premiums, compared with 12% for drugs. Four years later, drugs, at 15.5%, exceeded the hospital share at 14.8%. Clearly, drugs have substituted for some hospital stays and dramatically shortened others.

As drug costs have rocketed skyward, governments and health insurers have sought ways to contain costs. Efforts under way in various jurisdictions include the following:

◇ A 4.5% price cut was imposed on drugs in the United Kingdom effective October 1, 1999, with a price freeze for the following fifteen months. The establishment of a new committee to examine the potential cost/ benefit impact of new drugs on the national health-care budget had increased the difficulty of getting new drugs on the market; the first drug to be thus reviewed, Glaxo's Relenza, was rejected on economic grounds.

◇ Spain is implementing a price cut on the 100 most prescribed drugs.

◇ The Italian government is evaluating the possibility of seeking rebates from industry.

◇ French pharmacists have agreed on new policies to increase the substitution of generic for brand-name drugs.

◇ Belgium is instituting a price cut and policies to increase the use of generic drugs.

Often, price regulation seems to be the first step toward controlling drug costs in nations where health care is publicly funded, followed by utilization management efforts. The concept of utilization management for drugs — often called pharmaceutical-benefit management — includes a range of approval and other methods.

What techniques work best for drug cost containment in a public- or private-insurer environment? In a recent study, Merrill Lynch developed the following breakout of a 20% to 30% total savings by technique used:

Drug Plan–Savings Techniques

Technique	Savings as % of Plan Spending
Prior Authorization	1–3%
Formulary Compliance	5 1/2% –8%
Reduced Duration of Therapy	1/2% –1%
Therapeutic Substitution	5–6%

Source: Merrill Lynch, *Global Pharmaceuticals Research Report*, December 7, 1999.

Note that the substitution of generic for brand-name drugs, called therapeutic substitution, is a powerful cost saver. So, too, is compliance with a formula — a list of approved cost-effective drugs.

Who Pays?

Another result of rising costs in the drug sector is a shift of financial responsibility from private insurers and government payers onto consumers, through cost sharing, deductibles, and other methods. Insurance coverage for pharmaceuticals varies widely from country to country, as the chart below shows. The emergent gaps are primarily in North America for low- and middle-income earners. Both Canada and the United States have allowed a heavy burden of drug costs to fall upon patients. In Canada, drug costs are divided about equally among governments, employers, and patients. In the United States, public drug plans cover only 25% of total drug costs. In Europe, public coverage ranges from a low of 41% in Denmark to over 90% in the United Kingdom and the Netherlands.

**Public Pharmaceutical-Insurance Coverage
in Selected OECD Nations, 1995**

Country	% of Population Covered	% of Individual Costs Covered
Netherlands	100	90.3
United Kingdom	100	90.0
Greece	100	74.0
Sweden	100	71.4
Italy	100	65.0
New Zealand	100	64.0
Norway	100	58.0
Australia	100	50.6*
Finland	100	45.0
Denmark	100	41.0

Public Pharmaceutical-Insurance Coverage, 1995 (cont'd)

Country	% of Population Covered	% of Individual Costs Covered
Switzerland	99.5	43.0
Spain	99.3	75.0
France	98.0	54.0
Germany	92.2	48.0
Ireland	40.0	61.0
Canada	44.0**	33.0
United States	12.0	25.0

* 1994
** Revised figure, using OECD and Crop Counseil 1995 data. As cited in S. Morgan, *Issues for Canadian Pharmaceutical Policy; Canada Health Action: Building on the Legacy.* Papers commissioned by the National Forum on Health, Volume 4. *Striking a Balance: Health Care Systems in Canada and Elsewhere* (Sainte-Foy, P.Q.: Health Canada, 1998), pp. 677–735.
Source: OECD Health Data, 1997.

Increasingly, it is the patient who pays for his or her own drugs. This burden is increasing most sharply in North America, where fragmented coverage allows huge cost shifting to consumers, particularly on new products. Both governments and employers are shifting the cost burden of new drugs on to the ultimate consumer.

New Business Models

The pharmaceutical industry is one of the most global businesses. The reach of major pharma companies is truly worldwide. New global trade arrangements, such as the General Agreement on Trade and Tariffs (GATT), have strong support from big drug companies. Yet even these giants are merging to achieve greater economies of scale. There are thousands of pharmaceutical companies in the world, and the largest are becoming even larger. The top thirty drug companies account for 65% of global revenue in this market.

The 1998 annual report of drug giant Hoechst Marion Roussel (HMR), which had at the time recently merged to form Aventis Corporation, describes the evolution of this fast-moving industry. Richard J. Markham, chairman of the Board and chief executive officer, captures the key developments in a few paragraphs with remarkable frankness:

During my more than twenty-five years in the pharma industry, companies have seized upon different strategies at various times to grow revenue and profits and to build value for their shareholders.

Two and one-half decades ago, it seemed a company had only to launch some products, field a sales force capable of promoting whatever differentiation those products could claim, and collect revenues from a prescribing system that was somewhat insensitive to price and value.

That began to change in the late 1980s and early 1990s with public and private efforts to contain health care costs around the world. No longer could strong sales forces assure pharmaceutical success. As a result, companies tried new strategies. Some merged with each other to get bigger. Some diversified and sought to capitalize on generic drugs or over-the-counter products. Some acquired parts of their own distribution channels, such as pharmacy benefit managers. These looked like good strategies at the time, but we have since seen some companies unwinding their side businesses and acknowledging that "bigger" may not be big enough. Certainly, for a company like HMR, perpetuating the sales of extremely broad, mature product lines is not enough to produce sustainable growth or superior profitability.

At the onset of the twenty-first century, we are focusing on one core strategy: Innovation. This is based on the recognition that a company's ability to create value for patients and the health-care system is what ultimately creates value for the company and its shareholders. Breakthroughs in value come from innovative new drugs that cure important diseases or bring new therapeutic approaches to the market.

The new paradigm demands that we be innovative in our business model, as well as in our creation of new products. In particular, we must look at activities not critical to drug innovation and question whether they are necessary — or whether it is necessary that we do them. The decision to focus on innovation may imply corollary decisions to exit non-core activities. In that spirit, HMR sold our fermentation plant in Frankfurt and divested some other bulk-ingredient production operations as well as other non-core businesses during 1998.

Contract Research Organizations

HMR's 1998 spin-off of its U.S. drug development and regulatory operations was the first outsourcing of its kind in the pharma industry. Contract research organizations (CROs) take over the management of clinical trials on behalf of drug companies. The HMR business unit was sold to a leading contract research organization, Quintiles Transitional Corp. HMR also outsources to Quintiles the overseeing of some new product clinical trials and late-stage development of new products. Contracting with others who have expertise in a particular area is more efficient and lets a pharma company focus its resources on its core businesses.

In the past twenty years, pharmaceutical companies have followed the lead of other industries (once again the example of automobile manufacturing suggests itself) and have gone from making everything in-house to making significant use of outsourcing. This trend has progressed to the point that very few parts of the drug development and commercialization process are now considered core competencies and ineligible for outsourcing. The size of the outsourcing CRO market for clinical development alone has gone from $3 billion (U.S.) in 1997 to almost $5 billion in 1999, and will climb to just short of $6 billion by 2002. Similar trends can be found for outsourcing basic and preclinical research and development; chemistry, manufacturing, and controls; and regulatory, pharmacology, and toxicology work. As more pharma companies outsource more functions, the CRO market will continue to grow.

What are the benefits of using CROs? At the most basic level, a CRO can be considered the "hired hand" of the pharma company. Using CROs allows a company to better manage and control its own costs. If the drug company hires additional clinical development personnel to conduct a clinical trial on a particular product under development and that project is delayed due to a regulatory issue, it is the pharma company that must bear the cost. Similarly, once the project is complete, it is up to the pharma company to reallocate the personnel (and retrain if necessary). Obviously, by using a CRO, the pharma company can transfer many of those costs and risks to a third party.

But a drug company can realize a great deal more from its relationship with a CRO, which can have specialized knowledge that the drug company cannot afford to develop in-house. For example, a company with an active research and development program in neurology is in somewhat of a bind if it makes a significant discovery in cardiology. A few years ago, the company would most likely have shelved a promising product in such a situation, because it would have been prohibitively expensive to develop the expertise in-house for an entirely new discipline. However, today, by making use of the services provided by CROs experienced in cardiology, the pharma company would probably outsource what it is not able to do on its own and still see the cardiology drug developed. If the clinical trials were successful, the company could even use a contract sales force to move its one cardiology product, since its own sales force would likely have a neurology focus. The use of the information and experience resident in CROs makes pharma companies that much stronger, quite beyond the issue of costs.

For biotechnology companies in the junior development stage, CROs are the great equalizers. They give small biotech companies access to the same expertise used by giant global pharma companies. The only thing required is money to pay the CRO. However, it is easier to raise money in capital markets for a product in late-stage clinical development than it is to hire the appropriate personnel and develop a new area of in-house expertise. Small biotech companies can piggyback on the outsourcing to CROs by "big pharma."

Skipping the Middle Man: A New Paradigm

Historically, prescription drugs have been promoted directly to physicians. Pharmaceutical manufacturers employed representatives, known as "detail men," to make known the details of the benefits of each drug to the physician. Samples were freely provided to induce physicians to try something new. My late father, a surgeon, counted among his best friends "Red" Kelly, the detail man for Merck-Frosst. They fished together and flooded the local rink at –40° so that we could play hockey. Growing up, we had all our ailments — whether toothaches or bruised shins — treated with the full range of Merck-Frosst samples; our medicine cabinet brimmed with 222s, 282s, and 292s.

Major pharmaceutical firms continue to employ well-paid, on-the-ground sales forces — although now, as the firms that employ them combine, the forces are merging. But one strong indicator of how forcefully the winds of change are blowing in the drug sector is the fact that the fastest-growing segment of the pharmaceutical industry in North America is a completely different form of marketing: direct-to-consumer drug advertising.

This potent new avenue for companies seeking to launch new drugs, or to re-launch existing ones, has seen a dramatic, rapid acceleration of spending. By 1999, spending on direct-to-consumer advertising had rocketed to $2 billion (U.S.) in the United States. This is an impressive figure in the context of the $7 billion (U.S.) spent in the same year to market drugs to physicians in their offices.

This tendency to market directly to consumers is part of a larger trend in the drug industry to redirect its efforts toward end-user consumers and disease-state management. One phenomenon of the early 1990s U.S. drug industry was the trend for pharmaceutical companies to purchase pharmacy-benefits management companies. The first and largest of these purchases was Merck buying Medco Cost Containment. Merck paid (or, many say, overpaid) $6 billion (U.S.) for Medco, which had earnings of only $100 million. Similarly, other companies paid as much as 200 times the earnings for other pharmacy-benefits managers. Why?

To gain access to their extensive databases. Medco had data on 35 million American "lives" — that is, information on all of the drugs these people had consumed, and a significant amount of related diagnostic information as well.

To make disease-state management work, drug companies and others will need to reach past the present system, reorganizing it to the end user. Better informed consumers are one requirement for behaviour changes that will allow patients to derive the benefits from a fully organized care system. The patient benefit will result from interventions that are optimal in nature and appropriately timed to maximize benefits. Tighter management of chronic diseases such as diabetes and asthma especially has dramatic benefits for patients. At the top of the list is better compliance — that is, taking drugs in the right dose at the right time.

The Chip Meets the Drug Plan

One of the most popular applications of chip-based digital technology is the processing of drug claims. Why the rush to automate this task? The Institute of Medicine in the United States estimates that 44,000 to 98,000 patients die each year from improper drug dosing, mislabelling, and confusion over drug names. The chance to reduce these accidental deaths is one important reason for interest in tracking drug management using reliable, fast computer technology.

My own experience in the early 1990s as Ontario's Deputy Minister of Health is instructive. The ministry's $17 billion (CDN) budget included $1.2 billion for the Ontario Drug Benefit program (ODB). In fact, the ODB was one of the largest drug plans in North America. Two events galvanized my interest in automating this plan.

The first was a report from a coalition of senior citizens. It argued that thousands of Ontario seniors were admitted to hospital as a result of drug interactions, and concluded that hundreds of unnecessary deaths resulted from harmful drug combinations. These deaths and illnesses were not the work of murderous doctors, but the accidental consequence of multiple medications. Sometimes these medications were prescribed by separate doctors, each unaware of the other medications prescribed. In other cases, one doctor prescribed multiple drugs without proper records. The consequence for the patient was the same: two or more drugs combined to cause adverse, even lethal, side-effects.

If the tragic reality of seniors made ill by a program designed to help them was not enough, a visit from the RCMP provided a second strong reason. An investigation into the illegal sale of legal drugs had led the RCMP to conclude that fraud of the ODB represented a major source of underground drugs. Just how easy a target the ODB was became apparent as the RCMP officers explained their findings. An energetic and dishonest person eligible for ODB could visit numerous doctors on the same day (each visit, of course, paid for by the Ontario taxpayer). At each appointment, by alleging the appropriate symptoms, the fraud artist could receive a prescription, usually for pain. Then, after a tour of local pharma-.cies, the imposter could end up with as many as fifty filled prescriptions — and all the bills would go to the ODB. By the time the paper records were reconciled, the drug thief would have sold his illegal prescriptions.

And so, concerned by both adverse health outcomes and serious fraud, I turned to the best and brightest of my colleagues in the ministry for ideas. We quickly recognized that our answer lay in linking all 2,500 Ontario pharmacies electronically. By wiring all of the pharmacies to a central database so that they could share information in real time, we could improve the safety of patients and make fraud more difficult.

The Ontario Cabinet approved the "wiring" of the ODB, at a cost of $70 million (CDN) — which was recovered in a few years. Greenshields, a not-for-profit claims processor, was contracted to operate the network. Their efforts have saved hundreds of millions of dollars and many lives.

No wonder the managers of drug plans view the silicon chip as their ally in the struggle for optimal therapy, safety, and cost-effectiveness.

New Drugs, New Challenges

Public expectations, as I discussed in Chapter 2, are changing all aspects of health care — and the drug industry is no exception. An excellent demonstration of this phenomenon is the case of sildenafil, better known as Viagra, an effective treatment for male erectile dysfunction (ED). Its rapid rise to popularity has sparked a worldwide debate about the appropriateness and affordability of its use. While it is clearly an appropriate treatment for ED, Viagra is also immensely popular among men who are *not* suffering from any serious form of ED, but who believe it provides them with more virility. As a "lifestyle" drug, Viagra thus poses major challenges to health-care systems — and the people who pay for them.

In the United Kingdom, the government issued an "advice" to doctors in September of 1998 not to prescribe Viagra until further notice. By May 1999, the U.K. secretary of state for health had acknowledged that this directive was illegal. By July 1999, a new government directive had set in place a policy restricting the prescription of Viagra in certain diagnoses, and limiting how frequently it could be prescribed.

The cost factor galvanized British officials. With estimates ranging from 500,000 to 2 million potential patients in the country, and total cost estimates of £38 million to £128 million, the National Health Service feared severe cost pressure. Attempts to exclude all coverage of Viagra from the national health plan failed — after all, the National Health Service already paid for ED treatments that were less effective than Viagra.

Interestingly, similar kinds of initial restrictions regarding Viagra were imposed on physicians in the United States by a number of HMOs, including the large Kaiser Permanente. These, however, gave way to challenges in both the political and judicial arenas, leaving open the important question of how medicines such as Viagra will be funded in the future.

Conclusions

What does the future hold for the pharmaceutical sector? Drugs are likely to remain the main driving force in health care for another decade, when they may be replaced in this role by gene therapy. New drugs will continue to emerge from the laboratories of both the pharmaceutical industry and academic researchers. In 1999, U.S. spending on drug research and development reached $24 billion (U.S.). The tug of war between drug companies and the forces of cost containment will continue, gaining in ferocity. The stakes are immense.

Increasingly, drug companies will bypass physicians and market their new products directly to consumers. Pharmaceutical companies will become major advertisers on television and on the Internet; spaces previously occupied by tobacco and beer logos will be occupied by pitches for the latest miracle pharmaceutical product.

A new generation of computer chips will allow drug-benefit automation to go further still; your pharmacy will be linked to your home computer through the Internet. Prescriptions will become digital, and large amounts of information will come to you with your medication.

On the negative side, the cost burden on patients will continue to escalate. Governments may spend some of their late-twentieth-century revenue boom to cushion individuals against rising drug costs; overall, however, cost escalation will continue.

All four of the winds of change are evident in this sector. The financial squeeze pits cash-strapped payers against drug manufacturers; changing public expectations are leading the swing to a direct-to-consumer marketing approach; the impact of digital technology is evident in every pharmacy, every drug plan, and every research laboratory; and, finally, the new paradigm of viewing health as health status is the basis for a major thrust not only to vaccinate populations but also to spread quality-of-life-enhancing drugs such as Prozac and Viagra.

9

•

Public Health or the
Health of the Public?

*What matters in determining mortality and health in a society is
less the overall wealth of the society and more how evenly wealth
is distributed. The more equally wealth is distributed, the better
the health of that society.*

— EDITOR, *THE BRITISH MEDICAL JOURNAL* (1996)

A noisy, if nonviolent, battle is under way among various groups
within the broad spectrum of public and population health. At least
three camps can be discerned in this struggle for control of the public-
health domain. There are, first, the traditional public-health doctors,
who tend to advocate a separate and distinct public-health service with
sweeping powers of intervention to prevent the spread of infectious
diseases. Then there are health-promotion advocates, who are more

focused on public education and community action. Finally, there are the clinical epidemiologists, who focus on the health of the entire population and search for patterns of disease as a guide to how to direct resources.

All three groups, however, form part of one important trend: a movement toward more and more accurate measurement, aided by tools such as digital technology and population surveys.

What Do We Mean by "Healthy"?

One 1998 Canadian report, *Toward a Healthy Future*, prepared by health officials from both federal and provincial governments, identified a wide range of indicators of the health of Canadians, as shown in the table below. The study included measures ranging from self-assessments of general well-being to cancer death rates. The measure of potential years of life lost is particularly worth noting as an overall assessment of where increased efforts can achieve the most gain.

The list below is already long, but this type of list is in fact lengthening. Public-health advocates face an explosion of indicators and measures. As individuals, we have become obsessed with measuring our weight, body fat, and other measures of good health; similarly, as communities and as nations, we are engaged in a massive effort to pin down the exact level of health of our population with a raft of measurements.

Indicators of Population Health, Canada, 1998

Indicator	Measurement
Well-Being	
excellent health (self-rated)	25%
high self-esteem	49%
high mastery	21%
high sense of coherence	28%

Indicators of Population Health, Canada, 1998 (cont'd)

Indicator	Measurement
Function	
long-term activity limitation	16%
disability days (past 2 weeks)	0.85
very good health (functional status)	88%
Injuries	
injuries (admissions per 10,000 pop.)	72.2
work injuries (per 1,000 workers)	27.6
traffic deaths (per 100,000 pop.)	10.0
traffic injuries (per 100,000 pop.)	762.0
Miscellaneous Conditions	
low birth weight rate	5.8%
stillbirths (per 10,000 births)	65.4
overweight (age 20 to 64)	29%
Mental Health	
depression (probable)	4%
high chronic stress	26%
psychiatric hospitalization rate	709.1
high work stress	4%
Sexually Transmitted Diseases	
HIV positive tests	41,049
gonorrhea (per 100,000 pop.)	16.8
chlamydia (per 100,000 pop.)	114.8
Vaccine-Preventable Diseases	
measles (per 100,000 pop.)	1.1
pertussis (per 100,000 pop.)	18.0
Enteric, Foodborne, and Waterborne Diseases	
campylobacterosis (per 100,000 pop.)	42.7
salmonella (per 100,000 pop.)	22.0
giardiasis (per 100,000 pop.)	20.3
hepatitis A (per 100,000 pop.)	8.7
E. coli 0157 (per 100,000 pop.)	4.1

Indicators of Population Health, Canada, 1998 (cont'd)

Indicator	Measurement
Cancer (new cases per 100,000 pop.)	
women	346
men	501
Cancer (deaths per 100,000 pop.)	
women	151
men	232
Chronic Conditions (% reporting condition)	
arthritis/rheumatism	14%
asthma	7%
back problems	14%
food allergies	7%
non-food allergies	22%
Deaths (per 100,000 population)	
total	653
cancer (all)	185
lung cancer	49
breast cancer (women only)	29
cardiovascular disease	226
coronary heart disease	133
stroke	47
respiratory (all)	58
pneumonia/influenza	22
accidents (all)	43
suicide (all)	13
infant mortality (per 1,000 live births)	5.6
perinatal mortality rate (per 1,000 births)	6.7
early neonatal mortality rate (per 1,000 live births)	3.3
therapeutic abortions (per 100 live births)	18.7

Indicators of Population Health, Canada, 1998 (cont'd)

Indicator	Measurement
Potential Years of Life Lost (per 100,000 pop.), age standardized	
total	3,804
cancer	1,098
accidents	746
suicide	417
respiratory	113
heart disease	491
stroke	91
other	848
Life Expectancy at Birth (years)	
total	78.6
men	75.7
women	81.4
Education	
less than high school	35%
university completed	16%
Income	
average individual income	$25,196
low-income persons	20%
labour force participation rate	64.8%
unemployment rate	9.2%
Unpaid Household Activities	
any	89%
60+ hours	5%
unpaid child-care (some)	38%
unpaid senior-care (some)	17%
effective family functioning	92%
consistent parenting	58%
positive interaction	51%

Indicators of Population Health, Canada, 1998 (cont'd)

Indicator	Measurement
Smoking Bylaws/Bans	
smoking bylaws (population covered)	63%
smoke-free schools	65%
smoke-free daycares	51%
smoke-free health-care settings	29%
Personal Health Practices	
current smoker	28%
regular drinker	53%
14+ drinks per week	9%
5+ drinks per occasion	42%
driving after drinking (1+ times)	10%
currently using cannabis	7%
1+ illicit drugs, lifetime	24%
physically active	21%
walk to work	7%
always use bicycle helmet	29%
always insist on seat belt use	86%
took actions to improve health	47%
Health-Care Services	
influenza vaccination, ever	26%
Pap smear test, ever (age 18+)	87%
screening mammogram, past 2 years (age 50–69)	54%
blood pressure test, past year	71%
HIV/AIDS test, ever	15%
visits to health professional (1+)	93%
visits to a physician (1+)	81%
visits to a dentist, past year	62%
dental insurance	55%
eye examination, past year	42%
insurance for corrective lenses	47%

Indicators of Population Health, Canada, 1998 (cont'd)

Indicator	Measurement
medications used in past two days (1+)	63%
insurance for prescription medications	61%
unmet health-care needs	5%
emergency visits (per 1,000 pop.)	433.1
hospital (average days of stay)	11
health expenditures (% of GDP)	9.2%
per capita health expenditures	$2,512.72

Source: Health Canada. *Toward a Healthy Future*, 1998.

Taking Aim: Setting Targets for Public Health

Indicators are, however, by definition passive. The next step for those concerned with public health is to set targets for some of these measures — then set about trying to meet them. Here are some targets set by the United Kingdom in a document entitled *Health of the Nation*, issued by the British government in 1992. (Britain lagged behind efforts in New Zealand and the United States.) Note that the U.K. targets focus on exactly the same top six causes of premature deaths listed in the Canadian data above.

Health of the Nation Targets, United Kingdom, 1992

Goal	Target Rate and Time Frame
Reduction in deaths from coronary heart disease and stroke	40% by the year 2000
Reduction in deaths from breast cancer	25% by the year 2000
Reduction in deaths from lung cancer	30% in men and 15% in women by the year 2010
Reduction in the number of suicides	15% by the year 2000
Reduction in accidental deaths	33% among people under 15 and 25% among people 12–25 by the year 2005

The political dilemma of setting targets as opposed to listing indicators is that governments are vulnerable to criticism if they fail to reach targets. If, for example, a target such as "reducing breast cancer deaths by 25% by the year 2000" is not achieved, advocates are likely to demand more financial resources for patient care in breast cancer — and opposition parties will criticize the government for its failure. The positive side of this phenomenon is that greater action can sometimes be incited by the existence of an explicit target. The usual approach is to set targets far enough in the future to allow for a change in government.

An Example from the Bottom of the World

New Zealand has taken a thoughtful and thorough approach to the health of its 3.5 million residents. The 70 million sheep of New Zealand remain vulnerable to an array of perils including flash floods, but its humans are now the beneficiaries of a "health of the nation" effort.

The project began with a legislative definition of public health as "the health of all of the people of New Zealand or a community or section of such people." The next step was a selection of means to measure the health of its population, which follows fairly closely the choice indicators used in other nations. Then came the setting of goals and the development of strategies for improving public health.

New Zealand's 1997 "strategic direction" expanded on seven general goals supported by forty-one objectives and a hundred specific targets. The nature of the goals includes statements such as the following:

◇ to improve, promote, and protect the health of young people; and
◇ to ensure a social and physical environment that improves, promotes, and protects public health.

When it comes to meeting its objectives and targets, New Zealand's difficulty has been in gaining support for action within the health-care delivery sector, particularly doctors and hospitals. In late 1998, an Action for Health and Independence conference sought to engage the community and promote the integration of public-health goals with the health-care delivery system.

The New Zealand experience underscores the reality that it is easier to set national goals and targets than it is to achieve them. Part of the problem is that, while public-health policy tends to be set at a national level, actual health delivery remains a largely local endeavour, although, as discussed in Chapter 5, the emergence of regional health-care delivery organizations is slowly changing some aspects of this phenomenon. Only as larger health-delivery organizations embrace broader health goals will we see this gap bridged by commitment and action.

Apples to Apples: Comparing Public Health among Nations

In this age of globalization, nations are increasingly ranked against other nations in many areas, and health is no exception. The U.N. Development Program analysis uses a variety of measures to compare nations. This approach was introduced in 1990. Indicators included such measures of progress as life expectancy, education, and standard of living. As the chart below shows, Canada does well in the overall index but drops to tenth place on the Human Poverty Index, which places more emphasis on poverty and literacy.

Top Ten Nations in Two U.N. Rankings, 1995

Human Development Index* World Rank (1 = best)	Human Poverty Index** World Rank (1 = best)
1. Canada	1. Sweden
2. France	2. Netherlands
3. Norway	3. Germany
4. United States	4. Norway
5. Iceland	5. Italy
6. Finland	6. Finland
7. Netherlands	7. France

Top Ten Nations by Two U.N. Rankings, 1995 (cont'd)

Human Development Index* World Rank (1 = best)	Human Poverty Index** World Rank (1 = best)
8. Japan	8. Japan
9. New Zealand	9. Denmark
10. Sweden	10. Canada

* Out of 174 countries total.

** Out of 17 industrialized countries.

Source: United Nations Development Program, *Human Development Report*, 1998.

Even more bases for international comparisons are likely be developed in the near future, as nations seek to move beyond simple economic comparisons. Quality-of-life measurements are increasingly of interest as a balance to purely economic indicators such as the GNP.

Vaccines

Bill Gates, the wealthiest individual on earth, announced in late 1999 that he was donating $750 million (U.S.) toward global immunization initiatives. Why would the CEO of Microsoft sink such an enormous gift into this one initiative? The answer is, because he wants it to be effective.

Vaccination offers one of the truly great bargains in health spending. It is also one of the best items in the public-health toolkit. For every $1 (U.S.) spent on measles, mumps, and rubella vaccinations, more than $21 is saved in direct medical-care costs; for every $1 spent on diphtheria, tetanus, and pertussis vaccinations, more than $30 is saved; and for every $1 spent on polio vaccination, the savings are $6. And that's pure dollar accounting — the savings in human suffering are immeasurable.

Since 1974, the WHO and UNICEF have achieved a near miracle. Its expanded Program on Immunization reaches 80% of the children in the poorest nations on earth. These children receive immunizations against six key diseases: measles, diphtheria, polio, tetanus, tuberculosis, and pertussis (whooping cough).

In another worldwide victory, smallpox, once the scourge of children everywhere, has been completely eradicated. But the battle is not over. Current efforts in the area of vaccines include attempts to combat drug-resistant malaria, and, of course, the HIV/AIDS pandemic. Much remains to be done.

And there are still children in the world who do not have the benefits of vaccines. The global effort to immunize all children requires concerted action. Financial aid from Bill Gates, Ted Turner, and others among the super-rich is helpful, but only if programs exist to deliver the vaccine into the bodies of youngsters at risk. And immunization will not protect children from hunger, malnutrition, or the ravages of war. It will, however, allow them a chance to survive these perils.

Global Villages

As the winds of change continue to transform health care across the globe, the health of cities will gain particular importance. Our prospects for health in the global village of the future will be shaped by the increasing urbanization of the world's population. Huge, rapidly growing cities in the developing world will pose significant health challenges. The United Nations forecasts that by 2015, 60% of the world's population will be urban, compared with 45% now. From fourteen cities with populations of more than 10 million people each in 1994, we will have 22 cities of more than 20 million each by 2015. Health services have often been the responsibility of national or regional governments. Increasingly, local governments will be drawn into health issues. In particular, the major cities of the emerging economies of Asia and Latin America will face vast public-health issues caused by the poverty of their exploding numbers of residents.

Conclusions

For public health, the two most important challenges in the next century will be to put forward a global, health-of-the-planet vision while learning more about galvanizing local action.

A few more predictions, based on current trends:

◇ As the world's population concentrates more and more in vast, complex cities, the prospects for health will turn heavily on investments in sanitation. There will exist the potential for urban health catastrophes as well as the potential for profound improvements.

◇ Vaccination, one of the world's most successful public-health strategies, needs to be accompanied by broader measures.

◇ The movement to measurable indicators of population health is still in its early, enthusiastic stages.

As our measurement capabilities improve, the next challenge will be how to match local action to regional and national goals. Chapter 12 describes the example of the early experience of the Edmonton regional health authority tackling this gap at the frontlines.

A two-page ad in the January 2000 *Economist* noted that the Bill and Melinda Gates Foundation has donated $500 million (U.S.) to complete the worldwide eradication of polio. The Gates donation comes at the end of a decade-long campaign by the World Health Organization supported by the Worldwide Rotarians, which has eliminated polio in most regions. Whatever happens in wealthy nations such as Canada, the full benefits and potential of public health worldwide will only be realized with significant public-health investment in the developing nations; there is still plenty of scope for Bill to be a public-health Robin Hood.

10

•

Care in the Home

Patients in the 'hospital at home' program required eight days of treatment compared with 14.5 days for those treated in hospital.
— DR. ANDREW WILSON, *THE BRITISH MEDICAL JOURNAL* (1999)

Home care is as old as health care itself. Yet the home-care sector is feeling the winds of change as much as any. Modern technology allows many scenes that once took place only in the hallowed halls of hospitals and labs to be done in the home: diabetics monitor their own glucose levels; cardiac patients measure their own heartbeats. Remote monitoring and remote sensing are emerging as viable approaches to some kinds of conditions. "Hospital in the home" programs are being piloted in England and Canada. There are even home-dialysis pilot projects under way in some jurisdictions.

Caring for sick people in their homes is not a new concept. Informal, unpaid home care from family members has been around since the beginning of human societies. The shift to home care provided by a paid, professional work force, however, is a relatively new phenomenon. As I have noted earlier, the trend across nations to keep hospital stays shorter and provide a greater emphasis on home care is progressing rapidly. The other important trend in this sector is a shift toward the professionalization of home care. The pyramid below gives an idea of the current relative importance of various models — the more formal options are at the top, perched on a much larger volume of unpaid care.

Models of Home Care

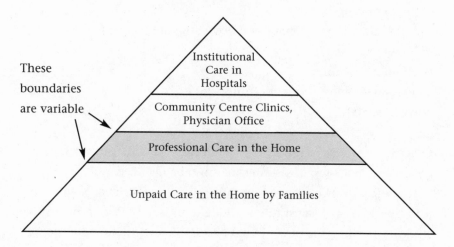

Caption content within image:
These boundaries are variable

Institutional Care in Hospitals

Community Centre Clinics, Physician Office

Professional Care in the Home

Unpaid Care in the Home by Families

The movement of women into the labour force has been a major force behind the need for paid, professional care in the home. The downsizing of acute-care hospitals is another. The bottom line is that more and more ill people are in their homes with fewer family caregivers to look after them. As a consequence, organizations that do offer professional home care have experienced steady growth and have seen an increase in the complexity of the needs of the patients they serve.

Defining Home Care

Home-care programs are defined as those specifically organized to coordinate and provide health care and supportive services to an individual in his or her place of residence. These services extend from clinical services to social support; they include, but are not limited to, the following:

◇ assessment and case management;

◇ Meals on Wheels;

◇ adult daycare;

◇ group homes;

◇ homemakers;

◇ home nursing care;

◇ community physiotherapy and occupational therapy;

◇ long-term care facilities;

◇ chronic-care units;

◇ assessment and treatment centres; and

◇ day hospitals.

Other services such as respite care, adult foster care, assistive device programs, and quick-response teams may also be included.

Home care can be viewed as three distinct models: as a substitute for acute care, as a substitute for long-term care, and as a preventive service. Of course, the three are not necessarily exclusive of one another, but coexist on a continuum. There is no universal model of home health-care delivery. In Canada, each province provides these services in a different way; other nations offer an even more varied array of approaches to care in the home.

Different National Experiences

In the United States, home health care became a growth industry during the late 1980s and 1990s. Driven by acute-care hospital consolidation and an increasing burden of chronic illness, between 1987 and 1994, investment in home care in the United States grew by $22 billion (U.S.) to an estimated $70 billion in the year 2000. In 1995, there were approximately 500 million home health-care visits in the United States, at an average cost of $90 per visit.

Home health-care services are provided by nurses; social workers; health-care aides; physical, occupational, and speech therapists; dietitians; and physicians, to name just some of the professionals involved in this sector. Nurses currently account for about 60% of all home health services delivered, however. For the most part, these services are provided by for-profit and nonprofit home-care agencies, although hospitals recently entered the home health-care market as well.

Sweden has developed a remarkable system of home health care. It can be provided in a private home, a group home, or a service house. (Service houses are unique to Sweden. They are used to house dependent people of any age, as well as elderly men and women who otherwise would not have suitable housing. The apartments are equipped with special alarms, rails in bathrooms, and other assistive devices needed to compensate for disabilities.) Home health care is provided by district primary health–care clinics. District nurses and nursing assistants are responsible for its delivery; other health-care professionals are employed as supporting consultants. Nurses' aides are available on a twenty-four-hour basis to visit homes, provide emergency services, administer medications, and provide general care services to home-based patients.

Public home-care expenditures in Canada reached $2.1 billion (CDN) in 1997/98 — an increase of $1.1 billion, or 104%, over the 1990/91 figure. As discussed in Chapter 4, this period was characterized by decreasing lengths of stay in acute-care hospitals and an increasing percentage of outpatient treatment arrangements; home care is an important component of the alternative models of health-care delivery being sought in the wake of fiscal constraints.

Mounting Evidence of Cost-Effectiveness

A number of recent studies in the United Kingdom and in Canada are documenting the better outcomes and greater cost-effectiveness of home care. Dr. Andrew Wilson led a U.K. study involving 199 patients with acute illnesses whose median age was 84. Half were looked after in hospital and the other half at home. The difference in cost of the two approaches was substantial; over a three-month period, the cost for the hospital patients averaged $11,425 versus only $8,875 for the home-care patients. At the end of three months, there were no important clinical differences in the health status of the two groups.

Not only was the cost of home care, even with twenty-four-hour-a-day nursing, less than 65% of the cost of hospital care daily, but the patients in home care were *less* likely to require readmission to hospital. These two findings demolish the two main objections usually voiced on the subject of home care: that outcomes would be worse, with re-admission rates higher, and that costs for intensive, round-the-clock home care would necessarily cost more than hospital care. Although many more studies are likely to be undertaken, the emerging evidence supports moving toward an even greater substitution of home care for hospital care.

Telehome Care

The application of telemedicine to home health care may become a key alternative to current models of health-care delivery, given the demographic realities of the next twenty to thirty years.

According to an Insight Research Corporation report, over 20% of U.S. home-care visits could make use of telemedical applications by the year 2001. The U.S. Balanced Budget Act of 1997 allocated the sum of $30 million (U.S.) for a "demonstration and evaluation project of telehealth homecare services for the elderly."

Telehome care has been measured against in-person home-care visits in several studies. A 1997 research project initiated by Kaiser Permanente, a U.S.-based health-care organization, found that telehome care allowed home-care nurses to "see" more patients in a day. It also decreased the visit time and ended up costing 33% to 50% less than traditional home-care visits. Researchers noted that with telehealth, a single patient could be seen many times in one day if necessary.

American TeleCare, a provider of telephone health care, initiated a telehome-care study in 1998. For fifteen patients, the rate of use of services and the associated costs were tracked, for the time periods before and after admission to the telehome-care service. The results indicated that patients with telehome care did not access as many health-care services, and their care cost less.

The silicon chip has, needless to say, also had a significant impact on home care. The current development of telehome care is a reflection of the increasing level of technological expertise in the telehealth industries as much as it is a product of market trends and an increasing social demand for economically viable professional services in a home-care setting. The wide range of vocabulary terms for the phenomenon testifies to its newness: "personal telemedicine," "telehealth home care," "telehome care," and "telecare" are used interchangeably. They all identify the use of electronic communication networks for two-way transfer of the data required for medical diagnosis, treatment, consultation, and/or health maintenance between a patient's residence and a health-care facility.

Telehome-care systems have an enormous capacity to enhance the delivery of home health care and thereby to lessen the economic burden of illness. The data chip has allowed the separation of information exchange from a physical visit. This separation is connected to a number of factors:

◇ reducing unnecessary visits to emergency rooms;
◇ reducing unscheduled visits to physicians' offices;
◇ providing early intervention or prevention of repeat hospitalization;
◇ teaching the patient how to manage early symptoms, thus avoiding the development of an acute pathological condition; and
◇ gathering information on vital signs' data fluctuations within a twenty-four-hour period, an important component of differential diagnosis and early prevention.

The potential applications of telemedicine in the home health-care sector include the following:

⬦ patient interview, history, review of systems, activities of daily living;
⬦ follow-up assessment for functional mental status;
⬦ intervention not requiring physical presence;
⬦ supervision of physicians' assistants and nurse practitioners;
⬦ consultation with nursing colleagues and auxiliary services (physical therapy and occupational therapy);
⬦ medical consultation;
⬦ medication compliance;
⬦ patient education;
⬦ facilitation of case management;
⬦ triage in lieu of transport to emergency room or office; and
⬦ monitoring of vital signs, electrocardiogram (ECG).

At present, telehealth applications are used mostly by people with chronic diseases such as heart disease, diabetes, hypertension, chronic obstructive pulmonary disease, septicemia, and adverse drug reactions. In this context, telehome care improves the quality of care by improving the access to care and by increasing the responsiveness of health-care facilities to changes in the vital signs of patients. This increase in the quality of care can be achieved even as the costs of care are reduced; telehome care can be delivered at approximately $25 to $35 (U.S.) per day in North America.

Not everyone is a candidate for telehome care. Patients need to have sufficient cognitive ability, hearing, and vision to use the system, or have an informal caregiver who can provide assistance. Their disease must be stable for this option to be safe. And telehome-care patients should have an initially positive attitude toward technology and be trained to use the system effectively.

Challenges to Telehome Care

Research shows that several issues currently represent challenges to the implementation of telehome care. These include reimbursement, liability, staff resistance, lack of standards, and client resistance.

Staff resistance at the supervising health-care facility was found to be one of the most significant barriers to the use of telehome-care video systems. A pilot telehome care project at Kaiser Permanente showed that staff regarded telemedical applications as a threat. Their major concern was that telehome-care systems would replace nurses and result in job losses. Nurses also worried that the new system would unfavourably change their relationships with patients. However, when staff observed how excited and interested patients were in the new method of delivering services, an atmosphere of acceptance developed. Nurses also found that the new technology allowed more flexibility in their daily schedules.

Telehome Care in Canada

Canadian telehome care is in its infancy. There are a few programs in different parts of the country that are starting to use information and telecommunication technologies to deliver home health care. The fact that some industry champions are emerging, despite the lack of specific funding for this area, is encouraging. There is the potential that knowledge centres will develop, which could contribute greatly to the dissemination of telehome care in the near future.

Only a few organizations are now involved in telehome-care projects, with a few more projects that are either in the final stages of planning or have submitted proposals for financing. These pilot programs, though not numerous, provide a good representation of the wide range of potential applications for telemedicine to home care — from monitoring pregnancies to emergency-room triage by phone to cardiac-patient monitoring.

Telehome care is catching on in Canada at a slow pace. This can be explained by the fact that the attention of many managers in the home-care health services has been focused on using information and telecommunication technologies to build an information infrastructure. Enabling the transmission of administrative and case-management information by qualified personnel, from the point of care to central databases and community health-information networks, has been the information-technology priority in home care.

While these applications are, strictly speaking, not a part of the tele-home care, they involve the same principles: applying distance data transmission to the home-care field. They thus represent a very important component of the emerging community-health information structure, and should not be overlooked. The chip is transforming the internal operation of home-care systems first; it will rapidly move on to transform patient care just as significantly.

In a presentation at the Insight press conference held in January 1997 in Toronto, Anne E. Becker, vice-president of Canadian operations for Olsten Health Services, reported that Olsten was using existing technology for telemedical management of high-risk pregnancies. The presentation identified three advances in home-care technology that will transform patients' homes into effective and efficient primary health-care sites:

◇ hand-held computers with case-management software for home health-care nurses;
◇ remote-controlled drug-delivery devices and dialysis equipment; and
◇ point-of-care diagnostics (e.g., X-rays transmitted in real time over a cellular modem).

In another pioneering Canadian program, two hospitals located in Moncton, New Brunswick, participated as pilot sites for an emergency triage service to address the growing demand for emergency-room services. The Telecare Pilot Project, staffed by emergency-room nurses, was receiving about ninety calls a day, after a year of operation, in 1996.

After the pilot stage was completed, the province of New Brunswick decided to offer Telecare as a provincial 1–800 service through a private-sector partner, Clinidata. Hospital telephone-information lines are not a new concept in Canada. However, the critical difference that makes the New Brunswick program more of a real telehealth service than just an info line is its use of software that provides diagnostic algorithms for more than 900 patient complaints. This makes nursing triage much more effective, and practically delivers primary diagnostic procedures over the telephone line.

Meanwhile, in Quebec, the InfoSanté (Info-Health) service operates out of that province's Centres locaux de services communautaires, which provide community health and social services. InfoSanté is a primary-care service offering, by means of a 1–800 number, telephone information and emergency diagnostic and triage services, similar to the New Brunswick Telecare project. With public-health services under stress, InfoSanté receives an increasing number of calls. In 1995, nurses answered 300,000 calls; by 1996, this number had reached 440,000.

One of the most well-established and advanced telehome-care programs is operated by TéléMedisys, a private-sector Canadian company operating from Montreal. It is supported by Medisys Health Group, Imasco Corporation, and Bell Canada. This company uses a proprietary palm-sized ECG device that allows cardiac patients to take their own ECG readings as soon as they feel any discomfort; they simply attach the twelve leads to the chest area, call the 1–800 number from anywhere in the country, and replay the ECG over the phone to waiting emergency/critical-care nurses.

The TéléMedisys program operates outside the Quebec public health-care system. The cost of the home cardiac-monitoring service for a patient is $49.95 (CDN) a month. According to TéléMedisys president Stephen Maislin, this service helps avoid 82% of unnecessary cardiac visits to emergency rooms for the company's clients. Another important benefit is the shortening of the medical response time. An average cardiac patient waits three and a half hours before an intervention; the TéléMedisys service shortens this time to twenty minutes. If it is determined that the patient is having a heart attack, the nurse taking the call can arrange an ambulance, call a hospital, and transfer the patient's medical record and ECG directly to the emergency room. TéléMedisys is currently monitoring 600 patients in Ontario and Quebec.

New Brunswick is undertaking a three-phase telecardiology project, which is a joint venture between NBTel Interactive and the Atlantic Health Sciences Corporation. The VITAL (Virtual Interactive Telehealth Assistance Link) project, which is led by a multi-disciplinary team of specialists from the New Brunswick Heart Centre, allows cardiologists, heart surgeons, and cardiology nurses to monitor a patient's condition in his or her home during the six-week postoperative period. Phase I provides hospital-to-hospital triage throughout the province. Phase II involves the initiation of telehome-care through the use of a device that looks "like a telephone with a small screen on it" and contains a digital processor. This unit allows the patient and physician to communicate, and gives the physician a means of monitoring the patient's vital signs.

One of the pioneers in the development of the informational backbone of home health care in Canada is the New Brunswick Extra-Mural Hospital. In 1993, the hospital piloted a clinical documentation/information system called PtCt (Patient Care Technologies) in one of its sixteen service-delivery units. The project was put on hold for a period of time when the management of the home-care program was transferred to the Region Hospital Corporations, but the PtCt project has been reactivated by the province. Once the system is in place it will provide a vehicle for multidisciplinary home-care teams to assess and record patient information at the point of care, as well as allow for integrating a patients' home-care and hospital information.

The Home Hospital

Dr. William Hogg and Dr. Jacques Lemelin, of the Faculty of Medicine, University of Ottawa, have proposed the creation of a "home hospital" in Canada's capital city. Their proposal for the Ottawa-Carleton Home Hospital describes it as an efficient alternative to traditional acute-care delivery. This project differs from the majority of telehome-care projects by projecting high-level physician involvement in the delivery of health services to patients at home. The proposed virtual hospital would include all diagnostic categories of disease with an average length of stay of four to five days of "inpatient" care. In the comfort of their homes, patients would receive daily visits from their physicians, "complemented by a multidisciplinary team of caregivers." The projected capacity of the home hospital is 387 "beds," at an estimated cost of $26 million (CDN). The project leaders anticipate savings of $190 per patient per day, "resulting from a reduction in staffing costs, laboratory tests, infrastructure, and fixed expenses." This would translate to savings of more than $26 million per year ($190 × 387 patients × 365 days), meaning the hospital would pay for itself within twelve months.

eCARE

St. Elizabeth Health Care is a nursing and home-care agency that provides services in the Toronto area as well as in several locations in eastern Ontario. Its dynamic chief executive, Shirlee Sharkey, is a leader in Canadian health care. Led by her vision, energy, and imagination, St. Elizabeth is taking new approaches to old problems in home care. This nonprofit organization provides a full range of electronically supported services for its patients: nurses have remote access to their patients' medical-record database at St. Elizabeth Health Care headquarters in Toronto, and can record assessment and intervention data while in a patient's home using Clinical Pathway software on laptop computers. They are also using PtCt, and can upload their updated records to the central database at the end of the day. Advanced technologies are providing St. Elizabeth Health Care with significant benefits, namely:

◇ standardized clinical care;
◇ a database with readily available information, which allows better decision making; and
◇ a competitive advantage in being able to access necessary information at the point of care.

St. Elizabeth is currently testing eCARE, a technology-based education and care management program. (The acronym stands for electronic coordination of activities, research, and education.) Based at an interactive Web site, this program uses secure Internet technology and an assessment tool to create individualized programs, enabling easy, high-speed information exchange among clients, family caregivers, and home-care nurses.

The initial phase of the project is designed for clients with diabetes. An individualized education program is created by eCARE for each of its clients, enabling them to obtain information specific to their own conditions and self-test their knowledge about diabetes. They can check their personalized home pages to find out, for example, when the nurse will next visit and what to expect during the visit. Clients can also monitor certain aspects of their conditions, and notify the nurse if an unscheduled visit is required. At any time, a nurse can log on to a client's site on the Internet to check his or her progress and monitor daily records.

Clients can connect with their nurses, with St. Elizabeth's Certified Diabetes Educator, and with other clients with diabetes who are using eCARE. The site also has links to other valuable diabetes-related resources.

Programs such as eCARE are changing the role of the nurse in response to the changing needs of consumers. Once, nurses were analogous to teachers; today they are engaged in a learning partnership with their clients, supporting them as they navigate the learning process and assume more management and control of their conditions.

The eCARE program also monitors clinical outcomes related to client care. It is a good example of how client-specific information in electronic format will help lead the way to better information management and make evidence-based practice more and more possible in health care.

Conclusions

From the cell phone to the personal computer to the Internet, digital technologies are allowing much more complex conditions to be managed at home. Meanwhile, better medications are allowing much more serious medical problems to be treated without hospitalization.

Care in the home, assisted by advanced technology, is *the* emerging phenomenon in health care. It is one part old wisdom — health care in the home, after all, is as old as the home itself. It is also two parts new technologies. I foresee that the positive results of evidence-based evaluations will cause health managers to assign a larger role to home care in the future.

How large a role will home care eventually play in the overall health system? Certainly a much greater one than today, when it represents only 2.5% of health spending. Along with drug spending, home-care spending is likely to lead all other aspects of health-care spending in growth; in fact, double-digit increases in home-care spending are likely to continue in most jurisdictions.

PART III •

Case Studies

11

•

Health American Style:
Managing Cost and Care

American political history shows that opportunities for substantial reform are few and far between. . . .

— Professor Ted Marmor, Yale School
of Management (1994)

For most of the twentieth century, U.S. health care was a "cost-plus" industry dominated by providers. The dramatic change in American health care is the emergence of new private-sector organizations that manage health-care costs. Despite their labels — "managed-care" or "health-maintenance" organizations — their primary activity in the 1990s has been cost containment. U.S. employers have been the driving force behind the movement to stem the rise of health-care spending, which gained real momentum after the failure of the Clinton health reforms in the mid-1990s. One of President Bill Clinton's goals, however — the consolidation of the industry into larger health organizations — has been achieved, albeit by the much less gentle hand of market forces.

Employers pay most of the health bills in the United States. They have chosen as instruments of savings market competition and the wielding of their enormous buying power. In city after city, provider organizations have merged and otherwise integrated their operations. Hospitals have combined with other hospitals as well as with physician clinics, nursing homes, and other health services. The new American health-care delivery organization is no longer a single hospital, but an integrated system.

Chapter 5 details the massive shift worldwide from inpatient to outpatient care, and from smaller to larger hospitals. This change is nowhere more pronounced than in the United States. From 1974 to 1996, the average length of stay in a U.S. hospital declined by 19%, from 7.7 to 6.2 days. Outpatient visits jumped by 57%. Outpatient surgeries, which accounted for 16.3% of all surgeries in 1980, had risen to 59.5% by 1996. Meanwhile, the total number of American hospitals, after peaking in 1974 at 7,174, has declined steadily ever since. By 1996, the figure was 6,201; nearly 1,000 U.S. hospitals had closed or merged in 20 years.

But the actual effects of managed care are more easily seen in real examples than in strings of numbers. In the following pages, I present a few U.S. case studies — stories of health-care organizations that have survived and even thrived in the age of managed care through mergers and embracing a broader concept of health-care delivery.

The Barnes-Jewish and Children's Hospital

Health consultants have dubbed the transformation of the Barnes Hospital in St. Louis, with its merger of a Jewish, a Catholic, and a non-denominational hospital, the "old God, new God, no God" merger. Certainly a great deal of faith was required by all parties to make a success of the venture.

First, a little background on the partners.

In 1914, Barnes Hospital was created with an $840,000 (U.S.) bequest from St. Louis businessman Robert A. Barnes. Since its inception, it has been the site of a number of medical breakthroughs, including the administering of insulin to control diabetes in 1920, the first removal of an entire lung in 1933, and the first bilateral lung transplant in 1989. The hospital has pioneered many clinical treatments and procedures that have been adopted as standards in such specialties as transplantation, cardiology, ophthamology, endrocrinology, neurology, neurosurgery, plastic and reconstructive surgery, and cancer.

In 1900, St. Louis's Jewish community opened the Jewish Hospital of St. Louis on Delmar Boulevard, with a commitment to providing health care to patients of all races and creeds. That same year, the hospital started the Jewish School of Nursing. In 1919, the hospital began its now nationally recognized research program. The hospital moved in 1922 to Kingshighway Boulevard, and expanded to 500 beds in 1954. The Jewish Hospital and the Washington University School of Medicine began their affiliation in 1963, making the hospital a major medical teaching facility.

In early 1996, Barnes Hospital and the Jewish Hospital of St. Louis formally merged to create Barnes-Jewish Hospital, shifting their direction from competition and toward collaboration. Each institution, however, retained its identity. By pooling resources, the hospitals have eliminated duplication, reduced costs, and increased overall efficiencies. Reductions in management overhead and improved purchasing power are two examples of this shift.

Barnes Hospital has consistently been named among the top ten medical centres in the United States by *U.S. News and World Report* and by physicians nationwide. Jewish Hospital's research program ranks among the national leaders for private institutions in funding from the National Institutes of Health. In June 1993, Barnes-Jewish joined with Christian Health Services, and the three became the charter members of the BJC Health System. The system expanded further in 1994 with the addition of Missouri Baptist Healthcare System/Missouri Baptist Medical Center and St. Louis Children's Hospital. Missouri Baptist, located in west St. Louis County, added greater geographic scope and clinical excellence to the system. With the acquisition of a children's hospital, BJC rounded out its continuum of care. Finally, the BJC system remains affiliated with Washington University Medical Center's hospitals and clinical departments, which are ranked among the finest in the world.

Two other noteworthy features of the BJC system are the Mallinkrodt Institute of Radiology, now a part of Barnes-Jewish Hospital, which provides state-of-the-art imaging capabilities — MRI, CT, radionuclide imaging, and PET (positron emission tomography imaging) — and also promotes an active research program, and the Imaging Center, one of the world's largest centers for the collaborative studies of brain structure and function, nuclear medicine, computer imaging, and neuropsychology.

BJC's system is one of the largest integrated health systems in the country having an academic medical center at its core. The innovative clinical programs being initiated in BJC help secure the clinical future of the medical school and training program in neurological surgery. The very scale of the organization will also likely buffer it from some of the financial pressures that are endangering some smaller academic institutions.

In recent years, the Washington University Medical Center has seen unprecedented growth, including the construction of new buildings, the restoration of others, and the creation of a network of pedestrian bridges connecting the campus. A state-of-the-art lecture hall and classroom building, the education centre is the focal point for the combined continuing education programs within the Washington University Medical Center.

The merger of Barnes-Jewish into a new, integrated system is typical of the transformation under way among American hospitals. Across the American hospital landscape, hundreds of mergers are leading to a consolidation of single-site hospitals into larger, multi-site organizations.

Duke University Medical Center

For more than sixty-five years, the Duke University Medical Center has been a source of healing and caring for patients from all over North

Carolina, the American Southeast, and the world. Year after year, it is ranked by *U.S. News and World Report* as one of the nation's top hospitals, and as the best in the South U.S.

Compared to many of its peers, Duke is a relatively young institution. Its medical centre has grown over the years from a small hospital and medical school devoted almost exclusively to patient care to a major medical centre with a national and international reputation. An integral part of the university, it is dedicated to teaching, research, and patient care, and also to helping solve societal problems.

Duke University Hospital, the patient-care component of Duke University Medical Center, is licensed for 1,124 beds, the third-largest teaching hospital in the country. In addition to the usual range of acute-care services, it houses outpatient clinics, inpatient units in psychiatry, a rehabilitation unit, a federally supported clinical research unit, and a diagnostic radiology suite.

At the Duke School of Medicine, student admission is extremely competitive. At the graduate level, Duke conducts a broad range of residency and clinical fellowship programs. In addition, the medical centre conducts a variety of education programs in the allied health professions, including a master's program in physical therapy, a physician's assistant program, a program in transfusion medicine, and a clinical laboratory-science program.

A *Time* magazine article in 1998 explained how the changes in the U.S. health-care system have affected Duke:

> As amazing as the medicine is, the money behind it is just as stunning. The medical center's total budget is $1.3 billion (U.S.) a year, and it has to come from somewhere. Not long ago, hospitals such as Duke relied on a neat juggling act: they would charge private insurers a little extra for a heart operation or a box of paper tissues and funnel the profit into all the extremely unprofitable things they do: teach students, do research, and treat the poor. It worked fine, until managed-care companies and government

cutbacks began shrinking those payments, and for-profit hospital chains started buying up community hospitals and competing for patients and revenues.

One of Duke's responses has been to cancel the planned expansion of its hospital, substituting a large ambulatory surgery centre. This shift is symbolic of the transformation of health services from bed-based inpatient services to outpatient and ambulatory services. The competitive pressures in the U.S. health marketplace have caused Duke to shift to a "lighter" mode of operations: length of stay in the hospital has been reduced, as has been the emphasis on bricks and mortar. In their place is a focus on better, faster ambulatory services — part of the new wave.

Helix Health

My description of the reengineering process of Helix Health borrows heavily from the work of colleagues at Computer Sciences Corporation (CSC) Healthcare (formerly APM, Inc.). Because reengineering was a strategy of thousands of North American hospitals in the 1990s, this classic example of the phenomenon is worth a careful review.

Located in Baltimore, Helix Health is now the largest health-care provider in Maryland. It is a diverse organization with more than 10,000 employees and 2,000 affiliated physicians and specialists, serving the 2.5 million people of the Baltimore area. The creation of Helix began in 1987, with the full-asset merger of two large hospitals in the region. By 1997, Helix Health comprised five community hospitals, a for-profit physician organization, a nonprofit subsidiary with ambulatory services and long-term-care facilities, and a for-profit subsidiary including a medical billing company, pharmacies, and other businesses.

In 1994, the leadership at Helix Health had established a guiding vision for the organization: it would become one of the premier integrated-delivery systems in North America. By March of the following year, Helix determined that, if it were to emerge as a leading IDS, the time was right to begin a full-scale effort to simultaneously integrate and reengineer the operations of its five hospitals. Helix had already begun to change its management structure, identifying some corporate functions to be centralized: finance, marketing, and materials management. The system had developed strong leadership at the corporate level that was very committed to these reengineering and integration processes at the same time. It did not make sense to separate the two; reengineering the five hospitals individually would have meant missing the opportunity to take advantage of the system's economies of scale.

Beginning in November 1995, a steering committee, as well as project, design, and work teams were created, drawing equally from all five hospitals and across all disciplines, including the managerial, professional, and staff levels. This approach to building teams was crucial in order to ensure "buy-in" throughout the system, as well as to develop redesign models and processes that were created and driven from the bottom up, rather than imposed from above. This integrated-project team also provided a base on which Helix began to develop a new organizational culture, attitude, and energy that gradually took hold throughout the new integrated delivery system.

To kick off the integration and reengineering project, seven months were devoted to building an operating vision for Helix, identifying financial, operational, quality, and service goals for redesigning systems, and establishing a set of ground rules for recommending redesigned processes to the steering committee. A set of "core system values" was developed from the core values of each of the Helix hospitals.

Developing this vision of an integrated health system at Helix was a lengthy, yet important, exercise. Leadership, clinicians, and staff from throughout the five hospitals collaborated to define Helix's values and establish what factors were key to its success. The visioning process was valuable to the project for several reasons:

◇ The collaborative nature of the process engaged managers in the integration and reengineering project, illustrating from the beginning that decisions would not be imposed in a "top-down" fashion.
◇ The vision and values, once established, provided an anchor against

which to test the impact and appropriateness of redesign recommendations.
◇ "Champions" were identified during this process to promote the project throughout the organization.

Helix had initially determined that an expense reduction of $50 to $75 million (U.S.) was necessary to achieve the desired levels of profitability and accomplish its strategic objectives. To assess the feasibility of this target range, several benchmarking analyses were completed comparing Helix operations to other state and national health-care systems and hospitals; based on the results, the overall reductions were readjusted to a target of $65 to $80 million.

Helix also developed operational goals and financial targets for each of four major operating areas: patient care, auxiliary, general support, and administrative services. These goals focused upon the identification and recommendation of opportunities to standardize and integrate services across the health-care system, such as integrating case-management models, consolidating and standardizing purchasing, cross-training staff, pooling distribution and administration, and developing outcome/ satisfaction measures.

A design team was appointed to each of the four operating areas, and these created a number of work teams (pharmacy, facilities, admitting, etc.). At one point, there were eighty work teams across the system, building recommendations for redesigned work models and processes. Each recommendation presented by the design team to the steering committee had to include:

◇ a clear description of the new model for operations;
◇ a rigorous financial analysis of the potential impact on future costs for affected cost centres;
◇ a statement of the potential impact on the quality of service delivery, with supporting documentation;
◇ an analysis of the investment costs — capital, employee training, severance, etc.;

◇ a plan for implementing the recommendation; and

◇ signatures and comments from the stakeholders of the process — that is, the employees affected by the particular redesign.

The first, least complex areas to integrate and reengineer were administration and support services. Materials management was centralized across the sites into one system-level corporate-manager portfolio; a purchasing director remained at each hospital. Helix also centralized many of the finance functions to the system level, including strategy, marketing responsibilities, and the development of human resource policy. To ensure that each hospital did not lose its unique identity — and its ability to attract patients from local communities — Helix retained a CEO, a CFO, and VPs of patient care, support services, and medical affairs at each site.

While the management of most ancillary and support services areas (e.g., facility and materials management, medical records, and laundry) was consolidated at the system level, a few functions, including patient care, medical libraries, and volunteer services, were deemed to be best managed at the site level. Some ancillary departments, such as pharmacy and diagnostic imaging, erected a "matrix-management" model, with a system-level director to coordinate and oversee the policy and overall performance of the department, and site managers responsible for its day-to-day activities. In most cases, these site managers have a dual-reporting relationship — to both the system-level director and the appropriate vice president at the hospital site.

Integrating patient care across multiple sites was a more challenging task. Several of Helix's hospitals had previously undergone individual patient-care redesign projects, with varying degrees of success. For example, one of the hospitals had recently developed a particular patient-centred care model that was expensive to implement, as it required several million dollars' worth of renovations to the facility. This led to concerns that Helix would not be in a position to meet its cost-savings targets in the area of patient care, and that the other Helix facilities might be required to adopt the one hospital's more expensive model.

The Helix design team assessed and compared each hospital's redesign model and results. This internal benchmarking process enabled the team to identify which practices worked best and should be implemented across the system as they set out to design a patient-care model that would be specific to Helix. A blended model emerged from this process that combined the best practices of each component organization.

A multidisciplinary team, comprising members from across all five hospitals, collaboratively developed Helix's system-wide patient-care redesign: an integrated case-management team model, including a nurse case manager, a nurse specializing in utilization management, and a social worker. The team ensured that the case-management structure complied with the principles and outcomes that had been established for patient care. This model was designed for the inpatient setting; however, Helix anticipated expanding the model throughout the system's continuum of care.

Throughout the redesign and integration project, Helix was also redesigning its information systems. Team members from the information-system project sat at the same table with the operations and clinical redesign teams, to ensure that the new information systems would complement the redesigned operations and clinical models.

Helix leadership elected not to integrate clinical programs across the system. Five hospitals, each with its own level of resources, case-management programs, mix of medical specialties, and geographic spread, would have been extremely difficult to consolidate into one clinical model. Instead, Helix leadership developed a clinical effectiveness unit, which works with each of the hospitals and is accountable for clinical resource-management across the system.

The redesign of Helix's clinical processes was a focused effort aimed at achieving system-level change in selected clinical areas. The aim was to develop, at the system level, the capability to manage the risks associated with the high-cost diseases affecting key populations, such as acute myocardial conditions, hip fractures, and prostate disease.

Cost-savings targets were not set for the clinical process design work per se, since redesigned clinical processes make possible savings in such areas as patient care and ancillary and support services. The clinical redesign team included twenty individuals from across the system: ten members were physicians from different disciplines, and the remaining ten were a mix of leaders from pharmacy, nursing, and other operational areas. Goals and targets for clinical process design were defined in terms of length of stay and reductions in the use of ancillary services. The clinical design teams identified opportunities for operations-based savings, but the responsibility for designing and quantifying any potential savings remained with the teams redesigning the appropriate area.

The clinical-redesign teams worked closely with the patient-care teams to ensure that the new models for patient care and work flows would be a good fit with the new streamlined clinical decision-making processes.

The clinical process design focused on three major areas:

◇ The team developed clinical-practice guidelines, pathways, and outcome measures to support effective and efficient clinical decision making for diagnoses and procedures that use more resources than expected, and for ancillary services that are inconsistently and inefficiently used.
◇ Physician information and reporting were redesigned to provide doctors with data and practice information, so they could identify variations in clinical use, cost outcomes, and patient satisfaction.
◇ The development of disease management set the foundation for the effective management of high-cost, chronic-patient populations, such as those with congestive heart failure, HIV/AIDS sufferers, and geriatric patients.

Helix Health reached its goal of identifying savings targets of $65 to $80 million (U.S.). It subsequently implemented the redesigned models for patient care, support services, case management, ancillary services, and administration. Helix continues to implement and refine its information technology system-wide to support the redesigned operational and clinical processes.

As Maryland's largest integrated health-care delivery system, Helix Health manages a total of 2,393 beds, treats more than 64,000 inpatients and 525,000 outpatients yearly, and makes nearly 200,000 home health-care visits. Helix's specialties include open-heart surgery, cardiology, rehabilitation, and orthopedic surgery. Helix Health also includes BWHealth, a partnership with Medlantic Healthcare Group of Washington, D.C., which provides clinical services and access to physician groups for the growing metropolitan areas between Baltimore and Washington.

Helix provides sub-acute and long-term care through its freestanding and hospital-based locations. Its other businesses include home health-care services, hospice care, medical billing services, adult medical daycare, assisted living, retirement communities, and seniors' housing. Helix is affiliated with HelixCare, an independent physician organization with more than 675 doctors and delivery sites that are dispersed throughout the region. Helix also operates a free, twenty-four-hour patient-information line and referral service.

Lessons from Helix Health

"The model that is evolving is transforming Helix into the truly integrated health system in this region," observes Steven Cohen, vice president of operations for Helix. "We aim to operate efficiently, control costs, be managed-care friendly, exceed service and quality expectations — and through all this, improve the health of the communities we serve. That is why we're here."

Note Mr. Cohen's phrase "improve the health of the communities we serve." This attitude is the true distinction between old-style hospitals and new-style systems. One focuses on patients; the other focuses on the patient and the *community* — the fundamental shift in objectives that accompanies the transformation from hospital to health system.

Some valuable lessons for other organizations contemplating this shift can be taken from Helix's transformation.

◇ Develop a clear vision and set of values for the new integrated delivery system, and use them to drive the integration and redesign process. Taking the time up-front to engage management and staff in vision development may seem to slow things down; however, at the end of the day, this kind of process will achieve considerable stakeholder "buy-in" to the project. This "buy-in" can fuel the project and keep everything on track when, seven or eight months down the road, indecision, uncertainty, or fear arises within project teams or among other members of the organizations.

◇ At the outset of the redesign process, establish a small list — no more than eight or ten items — setting the parameters for design teams' decision making. These could include "go/no go" policies on outsourcing, consolidation, and patient-care levels. Such a list can help prevent indecision or conflict among teams later in the redesign process.

◇ Address the redesign of information systems early in the integration and reengineering process, and ensure that information-technology design teams are closely linked with operational and clinical-design teams.

◇ Establish centralized, system-wide decision making and leadership early in the process. The project's steering committee should include representatives from system- and site-level management and physician leaders. Ensure the support of the system CEO for the process.

◇ Maintain some key management positions and leadership at each site of the integrated system. This will help to ensure that each hospital retains its identity and its relationship with the community. This is particularly important when integrating a number of community hospitals, which draw their patients from local communities or neighbourhoods.

Columbia/HCA Healthcare Corp.

For a decade, Columbia/HCA Healthcare Corporation ranked as the most dramatic success story in health organization–building. From a standing start in 1986, the hospital chain grew to more than 300 hospitals with revenues of more than $20 billion (U.S.). The darling of Wall Street investors and bankers, Columbia/HCA was the market economy's answer to efficiencies in health care.

By 1997, Columbia/HCA was the largest hospital corporation in the world. Its announced primary objective: "to provide the community it serves with a comprehensive array of quality health services in the most cost-effective manner."

Columbia/HCA's share price reached $44 (U.S.) in January of 1997. It owned and operated more than 300 hospitals and health facilities in 36 U.S. states, and in the United Kingdom and Switzerland. These facilities consisted of hospitals, ambulatory surgery centres, psychiatric hospitals, and outpatient centres in radiation therapy, diagnostics, and rehabilitation.

But like Icarus in the Greek legend, Columbia/HCA flew too close to the sun. Its wings melted and it plummeted — although not fully to its death. In its rush to grow, the company had neglected the checks and balances necessary for a sustainable business; fraud charges related to Medicare billings proved to be its undoing. The consequence of this litigation stopped Columbia/HCA's growth and reversed the company's fortunes. By 1999, two executives faced prison sentences. The share price dropped from $44 to $17 (U.S.).

The great hospital/health growth machine became the "ungrowth" machine — Columbia shed one-third of its assets to appease bankers and investors. Management personnel were also shed, to distance the company from its previous fraudulent practices. Many assets, including those relating to home health, were divested.

Lessons from Columbia/HCA

What can we learn from this tale?

First and most important, it underscores the point that there are enormous advantages of scale in the management of hospitals. Some consulting colleagues of mine studied Columbia/HCA for a competitor in Florida. They started with the assumption that Columbia/HCA enjoyed a 30% cost advantage on its back-office functions (billing, supplies, etc.).

Their analysis found, however, that this advantage was actually 50%. Efficiencies fuelled Columbia/HCA's phenomenal growth — and spurred thousands of other hospitals, determined to avoid takeover by Columbia/ HCA, to seek efficiencies of their own through outsourcing, other mergers, and large purchasing alliances. Thus, Columbia/ HCA's leadership in the efficiency drive had a profound impact on the entire industry.

A second conclusion we can draw from the Columbia/HCA experience is that national, or even international, corporate organizations in health care are a viable form. For decades, pharmaceutical companies have been the dominant health firms with international reach. Now other health-care related organizations, including computer software and hospital management, are also going global. It seems likely that, in the future, American hospital management companies will find inventive ways to become "local," for example, through partnerships, in order to successfully enter health markets beyond the United States.

There is also, of course, the obvious lesson that cheaters never prosper. In American health care the temptation to cheat, particularly government programs, is strong. Successful health organizations need a strong, value-based culture of integrity to succeed.

Overall Lessons

What far-reaching lessons can be drawn from the stories of these four emerging American health systems?

First, it's easy to see a consistent growth pattern. Each of the systems was built by bringing together multiple hospitals — in Columbia/HCA's case, several hundred of them. The resulting new beast in each case was a multi-site hospital organization.

Second, the health services these systems offer go well beyond acute hospital care. These are comprehensive health system. Duke Medical Center, Helix, Columbia, and BJC Health System all see themselves as having broad-based missions that include non-acute and non-hospital services. There is a notable shift toward ambulatory surgery centres and outpatient facilities.

Third, emerging health systems seem to have a growth imperative. Like the mercantile empires of the last century, health-care systems seek growth to cover their overheads. Head-office costs need to be spread over larger and larger operations for efficiencies to be realized.

Success Factors

In my role as a health consultant, one of the most frequent questions I am asked by hospital boards is, "What are the success factors in creating a large, integrated health-care system?" The factors identified by consulting teams I have worked with, from looking at many different kinds of systems, are outlined in the table on the next page.

There do exist a number of "virtual" systems, ones lacking a unified governance structure, that nevertheless are recognized as successful. It is possible to make such a system succeed — but it is harder to do so than in circumstances in which all of the above factors are present. The greater the complexity of the governance and management structures, the greater the potential for unproductive conflict.

Conclusions

Where the Clinton health reforms failed, market forces have partly succeeded. The Clinton reforms sought to create larger, more efficient health organizations, and this goal is being achieved through managed-care organizations, primarily HMOs, which are forcing providers to consolidate. The key Clinton goal of extending health coverage to the tens of millions of uninsured and underinsured Americans will not, however, be achieved by market forces. Remove the necessary political will for some form of universal coverage, and the market will create larger, more efficient American health-care delivery systems to which access for those lacking adequate insurance coverage will be difficult. The American employer-based financing system lacks the solidarity principle that underlies the European sickness funds or Canada's tax-payer-financed universal system.

Integrated Delivery-System Structures: Critical Success Factors

Critical Success Factors	Rationale
Unified systems governance	• supports shift in focus to integrated system-wide strategy and shared objectives • guards against parochialism and simplifies decision making
Single management structure	• provides streamlined, consistent management focus with single level of accountabilities at system level • achieves economies of scale through shared system services • integrates business units into system structure
Dynamic, system-focused leadership	• ensures focus on system strategy, objectives, and performance • maximizes development of integrated delivery system
Physician leadership and involvement	• creates partnership between system/business units and physicians
Single resource–allocation system	• ensures appropriate financial, capital and human-resource allocation for system-wide benefits
Commitment to education mission	• ensures commitment of resources in support of key community programs

Source: APM, Inc., 1997.

Employers will continue to put pressure on health services–delivery organizations to achieve greater efficiencies. Further consolidation of hospitals into larger groups — either corporate hospital chains or virtual health organizations — will occur.

Mergers will also be driven by the need to capitalize and maintain first-class information technology systems. Kaiser Permanente, the largest U.S. HMO, is currently investing $1 billion (U.S.) in new systems. For an organization with 9 million members, this is an affordable investment. Increasing capital intensity helped drive the consolidation of the airline industry; the same forces will continue to drive the health industry into larger organizations.

The corporate hospital chain is a beast unique to the American health landscape. The share-capital structure of these corporations provides a means of financing rapid acquisitions; fuelled by equity capital from Wall Street, firms such as Columbia/HCA have taken ownership of hundreds of hospitals. After a period of consolidation, these companies are likely to resume their expansion. Who knows how large such a system can become?

The same powerful market forces that allowed large enterprises to be created in health care are also capable of unravelling those same businesses. A slowing of growth or a reduction in profits is swiftly punished by shareholders. Falling share prices lead, as the case of Columbia/HCA shows, to a shedding of assets. American health-care organizations are likely to continue to experience much market-driven turbulence in the coming years.

12

•

Canada:
A Tale of Regionalization

Canada's system of universal medical and hospital insurance, now known generically as medicare, is considered one of the best in the world. It has achieved high levels of health status with minimal restrictions on patients or providers, and enjoys wide public support. Like many other health-care systems, however, it faces increased challenges from changes in the social, political, and economic environment.

— RAISA DEBER AND SHARMILA MHATRE,
UNIVERSITY OF TORONTO (1992)

The Lalonde Report set new directions for health policy in Canada back in 1974 (see Chapter 1), yet little changed until the early 1990s. One reason for the slow pace of change is that health care is an area of provincial

Some Major Provincial Health Care–Related Studies and Reports, Canada, Late 1980s and Early 1990s

Alberta	*The Rainbow Report: Our Vision for Health* (1989)
New Brunswick	*Report of the Commission on Selected Health Care Programs* (1989)
Nova Scotia	*The Report of the Nova Scotia Royal Commission on Health Care: Towards a New Strategy* (1989)
Ontario Ministry of Health	• *Toward a Shared Direction for Health in Ontario* (Evans Report; 1987); • *Health for All Ontario: Report of the Panel on Health Goals for Ontario* (Spasoff Report; 1987); • *Health Promotion Matters in Ontario* (Podborski Report; 1987); and • *Deciding the Future of Our Health Care* (1989)
Ontario Premier's Council on Health Strategy	Established in response to the Evans, Spasoff, and Podborski reports: • *A Vision of Health: Health Goals for Ontario* (1989); • *From Vision to Action* (1989); • *Nurturing Health* (1991); and • *Local Decision Making for Health and Social Services* (1991)
Quebec	*Commission d'enquête sur les services de santé et les services sociaux* (1987)
Saskatchewan	*Future Directions for Health Care in Saskatchewan* (1990)

jurisdiction in Canada. A partial list of provincial task forces, royal commissions, and committees from the past fifteen years or so relating to health care is reproduced in the chart to the left.

All of these reports favoured a broader view of health; each province rediscovered the truth of the federal Lalonde Report's broader determinants of health in its own time.

The winds of change that have led to the rapid integration of health-care organizations in the United States (see Chapter 11) are also blowing in Canada. However, they are buffeting a health system with a very different, and largely public, financing model. While cost-containment pressures on the part of employers are driving a move to managed care in the United States, in Canada it is cash-strapped provincial governments that are leading a movement toward rationalizing costs.

The biggest trend resulting from this movement in Canada, in nine of the ten provinces, is regionalization. (This trend does not include Canada's largest province, Ontario, which is discussed separately below.) In 1990, there were more than 900 hospitals in Canada, mostly general hospitals, each located on a single physical site. As outlined in Chapter 5, each had its own board of directors, a global budget from the provincial government, and its own management, medical, and nursing staff, not to mention kitchens and laboratories. The total number of people working in health care in Canada is about 750,000, making it the largest employer in Canada — 5 times the size of the auto industry. For three decades (the 1950s through the 1980s), the major feature of Canadian health care had been the rapid growth in its funding. While costs rose, little structural change occurred in health-care delivery.

Governments in most provinces reached two conclusions in the 1990s: first, they had run out of money for new health spending. The federal government was cutting transfer payments; something had to change. Health spending represented over one-third of most provincial budgets; the provinces wanted more value for this money. Each province looked at its health system and decided there must be some economies possible through consolidation. Not surprisingly, a move toward larger health-care organizations appealed to the provincial governments.

The major trend in the delivery of health care is the shift of services to outpatient care. This rapid increase in home care and day surgery, together with shortened hospital stays, meant thousands of hospital beds had closed by 1995 (again, see Chapter 5). But in Canada, very few hospitals had actually closed. Provincial governments were very reluctant to close hospitals, because the Canadian public thinks of them as the main source of health care. Shutting them down could lead to public-relations nightmares. A typical small Saskatchewan hospital, for example, had twenty beds and two patients at any given time, and cost $750,000 (CDN) a year. Anybody who got seriously ill would go to the nearest regional centre. But this local hospital provided thirty jobs in a small town; it was politically difficult to close. So governments in most of the Canadian provinces created regional health boards, pushing down authority from the provincial health ministry and pulling it up from hospital boards. If hospitals were to be closed, it was these bodies that were to do it, not the provincial health ministers, who had to stand for reelection.

In the most complete regionalization scenarios, hospital boards have largely been eliminated. Instead, each regional board, ideally, is responsible for a given population, and is allocated a budget annually by the province. It must do two things with this money: treat illnesses through health-care services, including hospitals; and invest in keeping its population healthy.

Saskatchewan, which had 137 hospitals and 137 hospital boards, now has 30 health districts. There are four districts in Nova Scotia and five in Prince Edward Island. In New Brunswick, regionalization initially included only acute-care hospital services. In Saskatchewan and Alberta, it was much broader, and included both public health and long-term care.

Ontario: A Special Case

Ontario has regionalized its health *planning* through a system of district health councils. But the money still flows from the provincial government to individual hospitals and doctors.

Saskatchewan's 137 hospitals before regionalization worked out to about 1 for every 7,000 people. Ontario began the 1990s with 11 million people and 222 hospitals — about 1 hospital for every 50,000 people. Its scale was bigger, but its dilemma was the same.

In 1996, Duncan Sinclair, an intelligent and compassionate former dean of medicine at Queen's University, was named to the chair of Ontario's new Health Services Restructuring Commission. As such, he took on the thankless and controversial task of restructuring health services in Canada's largest province. Dr. Sinclair led the consolidation of Ontario hospitals that was set in motion by the Conservative government of Mike Harris. Phase I of that task was to study, and then restructure *by command*, the hospitals of Ontario.

The Health Services Restructuring Commission (HSRC) was given sweeping powers to bring about change. These are Dr. Sinclair's honest, direct comments on the process:

We began with hospitals because in April 1996, the government had put two major policy planks in place:

— The so-called "system" would be, at the least, stable financially over the succeeding four years, funded at no less than the then $17.4 billion–based budget of the Ministry of Health. Two years later, that funding is now in the $18 billion range. The "system" is stable financially. The "cut, cut, cut" rhetoric notwithstanding, the "system" is not being cut! The government's recent announcement of massive reinvestment in home and long-term care is clear evidence of that.

— Hospital budgets would be cut by some 18% over three years at a rate of –5%, –6% and –7%. The last installment of –7%, due in 1998/99, was subsequently deferred, pending analysis of just how much money could be safely taken out of the restructured hospital sector. The commission's data now support our belief that the total is more like 12% to 13% than 18%.

In any case, we began with hospitals because it was obvious that serious service disruptions would result if the then 220 public hospitals acted individually to produce the required 11% to 18% budgetary reductions. Phase I of the commission's work was, in part, intended to prevent such service reductions. However, the main objective of Phase I was to lay the foundation for a sensibly sized, rationalized, coordinated hospital sector, or subsystem. Hospitals organized in this way are essential to provide accessible, affordable services of very high quality. Such a sector, or subsystem, is also necessary to render hospitals capable of participating in, if not to lead or share leadership in, the development of a genuinely integrated, comprehensive health-services system. . . .

By governance, we mean that our cherished health-services "system" has to act like one. It has to be a system and march to the drum of a common vision and clearly defined mission. It must strive for publicly defined, achievable, measurable goals and objectives, and receive the benefit of evaluative "feedback," all products of good governance. That governance must be provided by the government, by elected representatives of the people of Ontario. One of the most serious, overarching, and long-standing problems affecting the so-called health-services system now is that it does not have effective governance. Like many governing bodies, our governments have put entirely too much of their efforts into trying (unsuccessfully) to manage or operate the "system" and altogether too little in providing it with leadership, the governance it lacks and badly needs.

By integration, we mean that the many elements of which a genuine system must be built must be organized to work together in a smoothly coordinated way. Each should provide the particular health and/or health-care service for which it is best suited, applying the relevant criteria, including accessibility, high quality, and cost-effectiveness, to determine suitability. But all elements should be integrated into a genuine system so that each part works well in support of all the other parts. We do not now have an effective health "system," using the word in its ordinary sense. We have to create one and integration is an essential process to get it done.

By devolution, we mean shifting a great deal more of the responsibility for managing health services to accountable organizations located close to and controlled by the very people who receive health services and those who provide them. Devolution is a noun meaning the delegation or deputation of work and power (especially by central government to local or regional bodies). Just as Parliament devolves work and power to the government and its ministries, so we in the commission believe it essential that the Ministry of Health do two things:

— take up the vital responsibility of providing effective governance to the putative health-services system; and
— devolve responsibility for the operation of the system (and for local policy-making) to bodies made up of representatives of local users and providers of health services. We do not believe these bodies should be the regional health authorities in vogue in other provinces of Canada. We believe they should be different bodies referred to as integrated health systems. We conceive these to be partnerships of all the providers necessary to provide a full spectrum of health and health-care services to meet the needs of a defined population. We conceive the governance of integrated health systems to be drawn from the population to serve, like the boards of hospitals or community-care access centres (in charge of home care). In our model, membership in integrated health systems will range from approximately 100,000 people at a minimum to an upper limit set only by the organization's capacity genuinely to befriend and represent its members and avoid becoming bureaucratically remote from them.
— We have now, in effect, a single, humongous (and distressingly ineffective), integrated health system in Ontario. Everyone who carries an Ontario Health Card is a member. It is too big and poorly organized for its size! The organization is bureaucratically

remote from and unfriendly to its members and also to those who provide its services. By devolution, we mean simply breaking the big organization down into smaller, more friendly, manageable operational parts and delegating to those affected the power and responsibility of managing their part so that it meets the particular needs of the people and communities it serves.

The HSRC's task is driven by the same three principles evident in other provinces and other nations. Ontario residents and taxpayers want a faster, higher-quality, and more appropriate health system. Phase I of the commission's work involved the consolidation of acute-care hospitals through mandate mergers and closures. Phase II, describing the health-care system of the future, will prove even more difficult.

Over the next decade, it will be fascinating to watch the evolution of Ontario's system, which is taking a path different from that of all the other Canadian provinces. What will be the result of Duncan Sinclair's careful work?

Edmonton's Capital Health: A Canadian Case Study

Alberta, a province with a population of 3 million, has as its capital the city of Edmonton — one of the most northerly and most wintry major cities in the world; it is hundreds of miles closer to the North Pole than Moscow. The 750,000 people of Edmonton were served for many years by fourteen acute-care hospitals. Under the structuring plan of the Ralph Klein Conservative government, these were all joined in 1994 to become one organization: the Capital Health Authority.

Alberta's health reforms took a very different path from Ontario's; before looking at Edmonton's case in detail, it is worth understanding the concepts underlying them. As in the rest of Canada's medicare system, hospitals in Alberta used to receive global budgets directly from the provincial government. However, the election of Premier Ralph Klein in 1992 marked a radical shift. Always an oil-driven, conservative province, under two previous premiers — Peter Lougheed and Don Getty

— Alberta had invested billions of dollars in health-care infrastructure. Premier Klein came into office on a ticket of radically restructuring government. Based on a political philosophy often compared with that of Newt Gingrich in the United States, Ralph Klein's "contract with Alberta" was to eliminate the budget deficit, then to move on to eliminate the government's entire debt. To do this, major changes needed to be made in health services, the largest category of expenditure in the provincial budget.

The magnitude of the "big squeeze" in Alberta's health spending is evident in the excerpt and table below from the Alberta Auditor General's Report of 1998/99. While the financial cutbacks in most jurisdictions consisted of *reducing the pace of spending growth*, in 1995/96, health spending in Alberta *dropped* by $200 (CDN) million, or about 5%. It did not regain the levels of 1994/95 for three more years.

The expenditure history of the Ministry of Health is as follows (unadjusted for inflation):

Year	$ billion
1994/95	3.9
1995/96	3.7
1996/97	3.8
1997/98	4.2
1998/99	4.4

In March 1999, the government planned provincial health spending to increase to $4.8 billion (CDN) for 1999/2000 (8.7% increase). About 64% of health-system funding for 1999/2000 will go to health authorities, 20% to fee-for-service health practitioners, and 16% for various provincial programs.

The major feature of the transformation of Alberta's health system beyond the scope of the cutbacks was a top-down, legislated regionalization of the system. Under the new structure, seventeen regional health authorities (RHAs) replaced more than two hundred separate boards and administrations. RHAs have assumed responsibility for hospitals, continuing-care facilities, and public-health programs. They deliver health services in a given region, and are intended to work closely with local communities. The establishment of RHAs has reduced administration costs by eliminating several levels of management.

The government retains responsibility for broad policy setting and for monitoring performance. RHAs are responsible for integrating health-care services, promoting and protecting health and assessing health needs.

Overall, the shift in Alberta from institutional to community-based care has sparked the establishment of community health centres. These centres are designed to address a wide range of basic health needs in one location. Community health centres provide palliative and psychiatric care, health promotion, short-stay procedures and day surgery, addiction counselling, and social services. Each centre reflects the needs and the demands of the community it serves.

There is also an increased emphasis on health promotion, based on the Lalonde Report's recognition that a primary function of a health system should be to keep people healthy, not just treat them when they become ill or injured. Programs such as the Child Safety Restraint Program and the Alberta Heart Health Project are designed to address health risks before they become medical problems.

Community health councils have been established at the local level, allowing residents an opportunity to be involved in influencing policy and shaping health services. These councils are made up of representatives of the community whose main function is to consult with the public to ensure their needs are being addressed.

Funding was significantly reduced across the system, with some targeted reinvestment in home care. Two new funding plans were introduced: a population-based services plan adjusted for age, sex, and economic status, and a province-wide services plan for complex services.

The restructuring of health-care service delivery in Alberta was accompanied by an increased emphasis on accountability and performance measurement.

This is the provincial context in which Edmonton's new health system, known as the Capital Health Authority, emerged and was crowned "Leader of the Pack" in the headline of an admiring article in the *Maclean's* magazine inaugural health report in June 1997. In a comparison of measures including outcomes, services provided, resources, appropriateness of care, and efficiency, Edmonton's Capital Health came out on top in a list of sixteen major centres across the country. This ranking used national data and a statistical expert to ensure objectivity.

Five years into the restructuring process, Canada's largest integrated academic/health system has become a Canadian success story. It has emerged as a model for other provinces at various stages along the road to health-care reform. Capital Health now has a budget of more than $1 billion (CDN), employs 16,000 Albertans, and engages the services of 1,800 physicians — the largest group practising within a single health authority in the country. It provides a full range of health-care services for the base population of 801,000 in its immediate jurisdiction, and is the primary referral centre for a vast area far beyond the city limits. Factoring in this referral population (from northern Alberta, northwestern Saskatchewan, northeastern British Columbia, the Yukon, and the Northwest Territories) increases the total population served by Capital Health to more than 1 million. On average, one of every three Capital Health patients comes from outside Edmonton. In specialized care areas, the ratio is even higher.

The first two years of Capital Health's existence were marked by great concern and turmoil in the community, with significant layoffs of personnel and consolidation of services. As it moved forward, Capital Health began producing its own quarterly report card for the population it serves.

Capital Health was given control of almost all health spending in the region: the budgets of all hospitals and community health centres, the monies for public health, etc. But there were two important exceptions to its sweep of governance and management. First, remuneration of doctors remained in the form of direct payments from the provincial treasury; second, payments under the Alberta Drug Plan also remained separate. (It will be intriguing to see whether the Capital Health Authority is ultimately successful in wrapping its arms around the entire envelope of health-care spending with the population it serves, or whether these two exceptions will remain.)

It is interesting to look at Capital Health's early investments. These include millions of dollars in information technology, an outsourcing of materials management, and tendering for laboratory and laundry services. In short, Capital Health is being managed as one large business, rather than each of the individual component parts being operated separately.

Sheila Weatherill, CEO of the Capital Health Authority, describes the progress of the transformation to date as follows:

Overall, Capital Health appears to be a regionalization success story. Its creation was certainly not without complications, however. The first year, especially, was very political and very tense. Across the region, there was a sense from each hospital that some hospitals/areas were getting gored a little more than others. Overall, the regionalization process was initially viewed as a top-down, centralized effort to achieve consolidation and savings across the region. This left little room for "individuality" and any influence from hospitals and other providers. Finally, Capital Health has established its own organizational culture, and has moved beyond the politics of the 1994/95 health-system regionalization.

Population Health

The experience of the Edmonton Capital Health Authority in the field of population health sheds important light on how other large health systems might tackle these issues as they become more of a focus, worldwide.

Capital Health adopted a formal "population-health framework," outlining its approach to the issue. It builds on a number of reports prepared by Capital Health's medical officer of health. In the following excerpt from one of these reports, *How Healthy Are We?* issued in September 1999, Dr. Gerry Predy concludes that residents of Edmonton are relatively healthy, but notes a series of health risks.

Low birth weight babies:

— Study after study shows that babies born with a low birth weight face a greater risk of health problems, not only when they're born, but also later in life.
— For the past ten years, there has been virtually no improvement in the rate of low birth weight babies in the Capital Health region.
— The three-year average for the Capital Health region for 1996 to 1998 was 6.3%. Comparative data for 1995 to 1997 show that the rate for the Capital Health region (6.2%) is lower than the rate for Calgary (6.7%) and just slightly higher than the provincial average of 6.1%.
— Women who smoke cigarettes and/or drink alcohol have an increased risk of having a low birth weight baby. And a woman who goes to prenatal classes is 40% less likely to have a low birth weight baby.

Births to teenage women:

— Since 1998, the rate of teenage women having babies has gone down, but teenage pregnancy is still a serious concern.
— For 1996 to 1998, 23 out of every 1,000 women between 15 and 19 years old had a baby. The rate of teen births varies across the region.
— Over the last 12 years, the rate of induced abortions in Alberta has gone up, reaching a peak of 12.7 per 1,000 women aged 15 to 49 in 1996 through 1997. The highest rate is for women between 20 and 24, followed by teens between 15 and 19.

Communicable diseases:

— We've successfully controlled the spread of many infectious diseases like polio. And the majority of children in the region are immunized for diseases like measles and whooping cough. But other communicable diseases continue to be a problem.

— The number of newly identified cases of hepatitis C continues to increase in the region. In 1998, over 1,200 new cases were identified, up from 1,000 in 1997. The most common risk factor for hepatitis C infection is injection drug use.

— The rate of new cases of tuberculosis in the region is higher than the Canadian average. In 1998, there were 65 new cases of TB. For 1994 through 1998, 70% of the TB cases involved people coming to the region from other countries, and under 10% involved Aboriginal people.

— There were 75 new cases of HIV infection in 1998, the first year that HIV was a reportable disease. The most common age group for new cases of HIV is between 25 and 29 years, and the most common risk factor is injection drug use.

For each health risk identified, a strategy was developed, including actions for individuals and steps for Capital Health. For example, plans to address the issues outlined in the excerpt above included advice on diet and behaviour as well as more formal immunization targets.

Capital Health set three priorities in the population health area in 1998: heart disease and stroke, injury, and aging. Here is Dr. Predy's progress report from 1999.

Time for an update!

... For each of the priorities [set in 1998], work is under way to develop a set of strategies for Capital Health that will address these priority areas through a population-health approach. While it will take time to see significant changes in these priority areas, here is the latest information.

— Heart disease and stroke continue to be major causes of death, but the rates appear to be declining.

— Higher rates of heart disease in low-income people continue to be a concern.

— Injury rates continue to be high. In 1998, there were over 7,600 emergency visits for children under 19 because of falls.

— The number of hospital admissions for severe injuries continues to increase. Over half of the hospital admissions were for motor vehicle collisions, 23% were due to falls, 8% due to violence between people, and 4% were [for] self-inflicted [injuries].

— Although we're not seeing the impact yet, the population in the region is getting older. By 2011, estimates are that 10% of people aged 65 to 74 will need help with activities of daily living, and 22% of people over 85 will need help. Steps need to be taken today to encourage people to live healthier lives and prevent disabilities in the future.

The University of Alberta Hospitals Restructuring

Well before the Klein government announced its regionalization plan for the province in mid-1994, the University of Alberta Hospitals (UAH) had embarked on a major restructuring. An 800-bed academic medical centre located in Edmonton, the UAH was already reworking its integrated clinical resource–management systems, as well as operations engagement, in 1993/94. Its redesign phase began in March 1994, with financial targets of $40 to $50 million (CDN) on a cost base of $260 million, or approximately 15% to 20% of annual operating expenses.

In addition to reducing costs, the project was designed to maintain or enhance the quality of care for patients and the quality of the work environment for employees. Various design teams were put in place. Six patient-care design teams focused on redesigning the clinical course of care, from pre- through post-hospital activities, to shorten lengths of stay and reduce ancillary-resource use. These teams created care maps and clinical-practice guidelines for various categories of patients, with significant opportunity for improved clinical-resource management. The goal was better patient care at a lower cost. Six other teams worked on redesigning more cost-effective supplier and service areas.

When the policy to regionalize health care in Alberta was announced in mid-1994, there was little the project team or UAH leadership could do to predict how the creation of the Edmonton CHA would "shake out" and what effect it might have on the reengineering project. It was clear that the regionalization process was proceeding very quickly — the authorities were generally announced and implemented within six months.

The UAH project leadership was concerned that changing any major aspects of the project could slow the redesign process, distract the focus of the design teams from their clear targets, and affect the project and hospital staff negatively. So they decided to simply increase their original savings targets and proceed with the restructuring project as planned. The aim was to:

◇ reduce the risk of having control of the project and its implementation pulled away from UAH's own leadership; and
◇ position the UAH project to serve as a "model" for the regional health authority in terms of patient-care redesign, cost-savings strategies, etc. (This was important, as there were other hospitals in the region, such as the Royal Alexandra Hospital, that were simultaneously involved in the process of a patient care–redesign initiative.)

Soon afterward, the CHA became operational — just as the UAH project was entering its implementation stage. At this point, most of the UAH project implementation was halted. The lion's share of the redesigned areas — pharmacy, laboratory and diagnostics, materials management, and operating-room schedules — had significant regional implications, and the CHA leadership decided to determine region-wide needs from a top-down perspective before acting upon individual hospital redesigns. Also, the redesigned core processes from the UAH reengineering required significant reinvestment in capital, training, and implementation of its information technology. The CHA, which needed to pull 20% out of the regional budget within an eighteen-month time span, simply couldn't afford to build the infrastructure required to implement the complete UAH redesign. As a result, the only project areas to be implemented after the redesign phase were housekeeping, physical plant, and some administrative project areas.

However, after the dust had settled from the politics and shakeups of 1995, throughout 1996 and 1997, Capital Health dusted off the UAH project binder. Several of the redesign components were ultimately implemented on a regional basis, such as laboratory and radiology, the patient-care model (which decentralized management of hospital staff to program teams), and selected initiatives on purchasing. In 1997, a new "matrix" management structure was adopted for Capital Health and its hospitals. Each hospital now has a chief operating officer, who also has upper-management-level responsibilities within Capital Health. This approach seems to be working well.

Lessons from UAH

The UAH experience is an interesting example of how one organization can watch for potential opportunities to apply project-redesign models to a region-wide health system, which in turn can help position a hospital as a key player within the new structure.

Reengineering can enable individual providers to identify and develop their strengths, and therefore should not be disregarded for the sake of the regional-reform model. Careful management can determine which reengineering project recommendations from each hospital should be applied to the regional level.

Overall Lessons from Alberta

While the early evidence from regionalization experiences puts the process in a favourable light, there are areas where it has led to some valid concerns, particularly regarding the accountability and responsiveness of health services. In the 1998/99 Report of the Auditor General of Alberta, some of these concerns are outlined. The Auditor General makes it clear that the Minister of Health remains responsible and accountable for the health system's performance.

> Overall, the result of audit work continues to show that information and risk management are key to maintaining a cohesive and accountable health system. While progress is being made, systems still need to be advanced in order to better establish clear expectations, maintain budget control, and to measure and report results achieved for money spent. The following main points are aimed at achieving more cost-effective health services:
>
> — The risk is still present of delay in implementing authorized business plans for health authorities. The Joint Business Planning Group is to find ways of mitigating this risk and improving business planning. Until strategic direction and expectations are established in a timely manner, the accountability system will not work as well as intended.
> — The department is working on a strategic approach for performance reporting and determining priorities in business-planning expectations and performance measures. Analysis of annual reports indicates that a better link should be made between planned and actual performance reporting. Moreover, improvements in financial reporting can be made through consolidated reporting of health authorities and better use of financial analysis.
> — The risk of not meeting equipment requirements has been reduced by the issuance of new guidance to health authorities. However, the guidance may not be sufficient to ensure that an appropriate capital base is sustained for equipment.
> — The Department of Health is in the preliminary stages of establishing a stronger role in the coordinated planning of health facilities. The Ministry of Health should further develop systems

for planning health facilities on a provincial basis, notably acquiring information to support evidence-based forecasting of facility needs.

— The Department of Health needs to combine a high level of customer service with improved control over registration for health-care services. The system must keep pace with increasing transactions while demonstrating that registration is provided only to eligible persons.

— Improvements to physician funding systems are in progress with results yet to be demonstrated. The department needs to establish a method for measuring how much of a variance in the medical-services budget should be covered by increased funding. Also, the department should establish a process for assessing the benefits and cost of issuing clinical practice guidelines.

— The Wellness Project Office should continue developing systems of accountability so as to manage risks, maximize the prospect of meeting expectations within budget, and to render accountability for results achieved with the costs incurred.

Conclusions

The appeal of regionalization to Canadian health-care policy makers is twofold. First, by pulling together authority that had been diffused through a wide array of provider boards, efficiencies can be achieved without hurting, and perhaps while enhancing, clinical care. Second, devolving authority from the health ministry to a new entity at an intermediary level between payer and provider promises both managerial and political benefits: the regional entity can realize efficiencies by managing a larger envelope of funds, and the government is not seen by the public as responsible for the pain of layoffs and other difficulties associated with change.

A more long-term goal of health planners is to harness the power of the regional health authorities to improve population health. Over time, more of these entities will have a dual mandate of managing care services and improving the health of the defined geographic population they serve. Capital Health is one example of a regional organization that is already turning its attention to this area.

Overall, Alberta's health reforms have succeeded. But there have been difficulties, especially in the areas of:

◇ downsizing, restructuring, and reforming at the same time;
◇ finding the right number of regions for the province (there are currently too many, which leads smaller regions to depend on larger regions);
◇ involving physicians more thoroughly in planning change;
◇ finding the right leadership structure; and
◇ finding the right service distribution (the right mix of services and locations).

Change in Canada's health-care system continues to be controversial and turbulent. One of the few certainties is that larger health-delivery systems are emerging. Integration opportunities increase with the scope of regionalization, as shown in the following diagram.

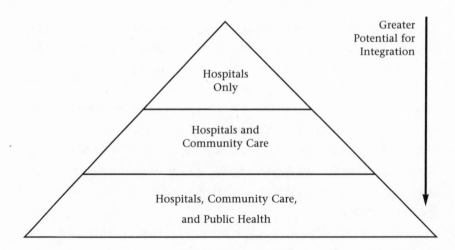

As Canada's debate over the future of health care evolves, the issues at its core are changing. The question of whether or not to regionalize health services has been answered in the affirmative. The new question is how best to manage these regionalized health services to meet consumer demands. Answering this challenge will try the talents of Canadian health managers and political leaders. In Canada, politicians rarely win elections on health issues, but they can easily lose on them!

13

•

Reformation Down Under

There is wide support for reform which would shift the focus away from providers and input to people and outcomes.
— ANDREW PODGER, SECRETARY, DEPARTMENT OF HEALTH AND
FAMILY SERVICES AUSTRALIA (MARCH 13, 1997)

D_o the same strong winds that buffet the Northern Hemisphere's health-care systems blow down under, in Australia and New Zealand? The answer is a resounding, if qualified, yes.

In New Zealand, the health system has been radically reformed several times in recent years. The Australian approach has been more gradual. Both nations' historic ties to Great Britain have shaped their approaches to health policy; the evolution of the National Health Service has been a key point of comparison for both New Zealand and

Australia, although neither nations' system mimics it precisely.

Significant differences exist between the health policies of Australia and New Zealand, but the experiences of the two nations share many of the same ideas, technologies, public expectations, and, of course, financial constraints.

To illustrate how the four forces of change have affected the systems down under, I will examine the situations of Australia's largest city, Sydney, and of its slightly smaller cousin, Melbourne, and finish with a brief discussion of the experience of South Auckland, New Zealand.

Case Study: Central Sydney Area Health Service

The Australian health service is modelled on the United Kingdom's National Health Service. The key difference is that Australia, like Canada, is a federation, with both a state and national governments. The Central Sydney Area Health Service (affectionately known as CSAHS, or just "Central Sydney"), which draws its mandate and funding from the government of the state of New South Wales, serves many of the 3 million people of Australia's most populous city, Sydney. The CSAHS mission is described in this excerpt from its 1998 annual report:

Central Sydney Area Health Service is committed to:

— working with people of Central Sydney to promote, protect, and maintain their level of well-being;
— fulfilling state-wide and national responsibilities to provide a high level of quality specialist services;
— providing, in conjunction with the tertiary education sector, professional health education and training; and
— encouraging and undertaking research.

The range of Central Sydney's facilities is broad. It extends from a division of population health to a nursing home, and from a leading teaching hospital to a dental hospital and family-care centre. The depth

177

of its family practice is unusual, with 500 family physician members.

Technological change and shifting public expectations are the driving forces behind recent innovations at Central Sydney. CEO Dr. Diana Horvath recounts some of her experiences of integration, Australian style, in the following excerpt from her paper, "Transition Crisis in Keystone Inner-City Teaching Health Service," which was presented to the 1997 King's Fund International Seminar in London, England:

From Troubled Hospital to Area Health System

... On December 24, 1992, I took over as CEO, formally appointed by the Governor-in-Council. There was not another member of the senior executive staff left; the Area office staff was thirteen strong; the Acting Board Chairman retired with metastatic lung cancer; the Auditor-General disclaimed the accounts (it took six months to determine the year-end cash result); and Australia started to close down for the Christmas/Summer holiday period. As well, the State and Federal governments had announced the transfer of the major Veterans' Affairs Hospital (Concord) to CSAHS on July 1, 1993.

At that time the main hospital was still hemorrhaging [money] at the rate of $1 million (Austral.) per month. It was necessary to close beds (75), reduce operating theatre sessions, reduce staff (500), and reduce activity by 10%.

By the end of calendar year 1993, the staff in the area facilities had been reduced by some 1,500 from 10,000; and a further $8 million had been paid off the accumulated debt. A clinical service plan had been developed to drive the integration of Concord as a second major general teaching hospital within Central Sydney.

A mental-health services plan was negotiated, between a set of warring parties, to progressively downsize a 450-bed psychiatric hospital while establishing acute-admission units in each of the general teaching hospitals and transferring clinical resources to community mental-health activities.

The opportunity was taken to extend the concept of clinical services planning to this site — and commence a process of identifying area-wide clinical services — with designation of area clinical directors who were empowered to negotiate the clinical changes necessary to drive the process.

What lessons can be learned?

The hospitals and their staff learned to trust all over again. The relationship with clinical and support staff alike remains frank and productive — as the process of microeconomic reform continues apace. There is a sense of progress and a feeling of anticipation in and around the campuses. The infrastructure is being progressively rationalized — fourteen kitchens have reduced to two. Accounting and payroll functions have been centralized for economies of scale, and competitive "best practices" established.

. . . Health services have the enormous advantage of being "good": intimate things done by people to people who trust them to help and not harm. Very few enterprises have such a satisfying, challenging, and personal appeal. I think it is a mistake to ignore or waste this precious focus; or to dissipate it through creating our own competitive assembly lines. There is nothing yet as inventive as the human mind when it is turned on.

Today, CSAHS is Australia's largest health service. It has established priorities in the four areas that cause 80% of premature deaths among the 460,000 residents it serves:

◇ cardiovascular disease;
◇ mental health;
◇ injury; and
◇ cancer.

As well, the nearly 9,000 staff members spend $793 million (Austral.) under their performance agreement with the state government of New South Wales. The range of health services provided covers the gamut from prevention to acute-care hospital services. Unlike the United Kingdom, the

Australian federation divides responsibility for health between the state and federal levels. The federal government plays a key role in paying doctors.

The story of Central Sydney's transformation over the past few years is told in the numbers of the table below.

Trends at Central Sydney, 1996–1999

Year	# of Inpatient Beds	Admissions per Annum	Bed Days per Annum	Average Length of Stay (Days)
1996/97	2,337	137,338	711,842	5.2
1997/98	2,189	136,512	681,973	5.0
1998/99	1,995	132,181	633,400	4.8

Source: Annual Reports, Central Sydney Health Service.

Lessons from Central Sydney

What can we learn from the story of Central Sydney and Dr. Horvath's experiences? First, that while the process of change in health organizations is traumatic and jarring, with good leadership, trust can be successfully restored among staff. Second, that Central Sydney faced many of the very same challenges we have seen again and again around the world: the reduction of beds, shortening of lengths of stay, and consequent staffing layoffs. In three years, Central Sydney saw a reduction of 341 beds, or about 15%. Patients' average length of stay shortened by about 8% over the same period.

It is hoped that there is an unlocking of human imagination and ingenuity in finding new ways of delivering care. In the Sydney example, determined leadership unlocked the potential of those in the organization to excel. The transformation of old-style, hierarchical command and control structures into newer, devolved-authority, team-based entities is only beginning in health. This direction has much promise for the future.

Case Study: Southern Health Care Network, Melbourne

In case after case, as we have seen, the response to the four winds is a drive to integrate care. The Southern Health Care Network (SHCN), based in Melbourne, Australia, is no exception; it is an example of an effort to achieve integration across a range of services for a population of 750,000. The key elements of SHCN include a large teaching hospital, two district general hospitals, a psychiatric hospital, a small, acute-rehabilitation hospital, and a service that provides care for the aged, including nursing homes and hostels.

SHCN has set four simple objectives for itself:

◇ improve access to care;
◇ improve continuity of care;
◇ improve effectiveness of care; and
◇ improve efficiency.

One focus of SHCN is to maximize the use of its existing infrastructure while moving toward a more integrated system of care.

The SHCN is building on a base of community health centres, which are already well established in the Melbourne suburbs and are oriented to delivering primary-care services. The community health services are being encouraged to join SHCN, which allows for greater integration of care.

SHCN has moved to a clinical program–management approach, which is described by the CEO as follows:

> To facilitate the involvement and commitment of [SHCN's] clinicians, it has reorganized the direct clinical staff of its hospitals into twelve clinical programs. This includes medical and nursing staff, and in the case of the mental health and aged care, allied health staff are also included. Clinical programs are also supported by clinical support (including intensive care, perio-operative services, imaging, pathology, acute rehabilitation, allied health and

pharmacy) and non-clinical support divisions, finance and information services, and corporate services.

Each clinical program is led by a "clinical partnership" including a program medical director, nursing director, and, in the case of mental health and aged care, an allied health director. A business manager, a senior general administrator with the training and experience equivalent to a mid-sized hospital chief executive, supports the partnership. Most business managers support a number of programs. Clinical partners are line responsible to the CEO, but this is used sparingly for "hiring and firing" level issues. Operational coordination is achieved through an internal service agreement, which is negotiated annually and covers revenue, cost and quality performance targets, specific projects, and reporting arrangements. An executive sponsor is allocated to each program to negotiate their service agreement, assist the program in achieving its service agreement through initiatives on their behalf on the executive and within the network, and to monitor performance on behalf of the CEO.

Like Duke University's medical centre, and many other emergent health systems, SHCN made plans to build a day-surgery centre. The network's literature describes the Cranbourne Integrated Care Centre, now under construction, as follows:

> This centre will provide day-surgery and day-procedure facilities, renal dialysis, specialist consulting rooms, pathology, imaging and pharmacy services, community mental health, community rehabilitation, and other aged-care services and community health with integration of services, including shared records. Other community-based service providers will collocate.

It was estimated that the Cranbourne Integrated Care Centre would cost $10 million (Austral.) to establish.

One interesting aspect of SHCN is its program of coordinated care trials for patients with very high acute-care costs. The idea is to better organize the care of these high-need patients, with the twin goals of lower costs and better patient outcomes.

The SHCN trials enrolled patients that ran up acute-care costs of over $4,000 (Austral.) in the previous two years, and are planned to be two years in length. Actuarial studies have determined that patients of the type recruited for these trials currently consume more than ten times as much hospital care, more than ten times as many pharmaceuticals, and more than seventeen times as much doctors' attention than the average patient, as measured by cost.

The trials will be organized as follows: each enrollee's Commonwealth Medical Benefits, pharmaceutical benefits, and estimated state public hospital costs, based on an actuarial assessment of predicted use over the next two years, will be pooled. This pool will then be used to fund the following:

◇ actual health services used by the enrollee;
◇ protocol-based care coordination and follow-up by general practitioner;
◇ service coordination, including case managers; and
◇ additional services if the pool has a surplus.

The trials will include 2,500 enrolled patients and 500 in a control sample. Evaluations of the system at the national and local levels are being separately funded to assess both the health status and the satisfaction level of the enrollees. This separate evaluation process reflects the tensions inherent in the involvement of both national and state governments in health care.

The trials are an effort to break down the existing funding silos and pool resources to focus on high-need patients more effectively. ("Funding silos" is a term used by health policy makers to describe the separation of funding according to the type of provider. Doctor budgets are in a separate silo from those for hospital or drug budgets, for example.)

Lessons from SHCN

The first observation is that a program model of management is replacing a long-standing approach based on medical specialties. Health systems are organizing services in a manner understandable to patients rather than on the history of medical disciplines. More integrated care is the clear goal.

Next, we can note yet more evidence of a lighter, faster, more cost-effective approach in this new world of health care, in which $10 million (Austral.) ambulatory facilities such as Cranbourne Integrated Care Centre displace $100 million hospitals.

It is too early to fully appreciate how the high-needs patient trials will turn out, but some lessons have already emerged. These include:

◇ the importance of the role of general practitioners, but also these practitioners' limited skill and knowledge base for assessing and arranging care coordination;
◇ the importance of information systems for transmitting patient-care information, but the limited availability of cost-effective ways to implement some systems;
◇ the difficulty of tracking patients and the inaccuracy of hospital databases;
◇ the lack of availability of care-coordination tools; and
◇ the impossibility of "rational" evaluation in complex field studies.

J.U. Stoelwinder, the CEO of the Southern Health Care Network, noted the similarities between Australian and American reforms in the following comments on SHCN, taken from his Toronto presentation to the Ontario Hospital Association in November 1997:

It seems inevitable to me that in Australia, as in many countries, the dominant neoconservative economic philosophy in public-sector service delivery will persist. If not a complete shift to privatization, there will be at least an effort to redesign funding for health care so that the financial risk shifts from the payer to the provider. The most evident way of achieving this is to increasingly aggregate funding and link payment to contractually defined outcomes. The end point of this is full capitation funding. The end point of capitation funding and hence the shift of risk to service providers is vertically integrated service-delivery organizations. This has happened under managed care in the United States. It is also the underlying assumption we have made in forming the Southern Health Care Network.

Mr. Stoelwinder goes on to suggest the fate of hospitals that do not become part of larger, more integrated systems of care.

As the requirement for hospital beds declines, hospitals can only get smaller or, to maintain critical size, they will need to get a larger market. If they are not integrated into a system of care covering their patients, they will become technical workshops, progressively disconnected from the real action — integrated care of good quality. It is for this reason that we are trying to reinvent our hospitals as part of, and supporting, a local system of care.

South Auckland Health

As the dynamic chief executive of South Auckland Health, a New Zealand Crown health enterprise, Lewis Levy set out to reshape a hospital system into a health system. How did this come about? The emergence of Crown health enterprises, or CHEs, in New Zealand, as discussed briefly in Chapter 1, had its roots in a radical swing in New Zealand's government — from the far-left government of David Lange with its aim of building a socialist utopia in the South Pacific, to its right-wing successor's fervent embrace of the market-driven economy.

In its efforts to create internal markets for health-care services and thus achieve dramatic improvements in efficiency, the government of New Zealand in 1993 created twenty-three CHEs. The shareholders were not private individuals or corporations, but the Ministry of Finance and the Ministry of Crown Enterprises. However, these Crown-held businesses were made to compete in obtaining revenue. New Zealand was divided into four regions, each with its own health authority controlling a set budget from the Ministry of Health. All twenty-three CHEs competed for this money on the basis of annual offerings of service. These proposals were the basis for contracts between the regional purchasers and each CHE to provide specific volumes of specific medical services. New Zealand represents an attempt, along with the Scandinavian countries and the United Kingdom, to bring the virtues of the market to bear without moving towards a fully privatized health system. The government's underlying hope was that competition among these enterprises would lead to both better and more cost-efficient health services.

Here, then, is the basic profile of one of these twenty-three hybrid entities, South Auckland Health, as noted in its own annual report:

Counties Manukau Health Limited, better known as South Auckland Health, is the major provider of public-health services to the communities of South and East Auckland.

South Auckland Health was established under the Health and Disability Services Act 1993, as one of three Crown health enterprises in the greater Auckland region.

The population served and the range and volume of services that South Auckland Health provides are determined by contracts predominantly with the purchaser of health and disability services in the northern region of the North Island (Northern Regional Health Authority).

The 1991 census indicates the current population served by South Auckland Health is 314,700, projected to increase to 344,400 (medium projection) by 1996, and 427,400 (medium projection) by 2006. . . . The provisional 1996 census indicates that the population of South Auckland has increased by 11.9% over the 1991 census, with a population now of 341,000.

The population served is characterized by a changing cultural mix, with the 1991 census indicating a current ethnic mix of 214,311 non-Maori and non-Pacific Island, 48,149 Pacific Island, and 52,240 Maori.

South Auckland Health provides a wide but not complete range of specialist secondary services and a selected range of community services, as well as the following niche specialist tertiary services:

— orthopedic surgery;
— plastic, reconstructive, and maxillofacial surgery;
— spinal injury rehabilitation;
— renal dialysis; and
— neonatal intensive care.

South Auckland Health is participating in the mental health deinstitutionalization programme which is led by North Health and coordinated by the Ministry of Health. This deinstitutionalization programme will result in the relocation of services for those patients requiring longer term rehabilitation and long-term care.

Middlemore Hospital currently operates 591 resourced beds and is predominantly an acute-service hospital, although significant amounts of elective services are also provided. Inpatient services are also provided at South Auckland Health's other facilities:

— Kingseat Hospital (until its closure in 1997) — 108 beds;
— Otara Spinal Rehabilitation Unit — 35 beds;
— Pukekohe Hospital — 36 beds;
— Franklin Memorial Hospital — 18 beds;
— Papakura Hospital — 14 beds; and
— Botany Downs Maternity Unit — 15 beds.

South Auckland Health provides a total of 817 resourced beds. Services are provided by 2,370 full-time equivalent staff.

Daypatients, outpatients and community services are provided at all the above facilities as well as through small community-based facilities distributed throughout the region. These services will predominantly be provided through the new community-based SuperClinics™ when they are commissioned in 1997.

In 1996, Mr. Levy, the CEO, took an optimistic view of the future, yet also identified some unresolved questions:

In a new, post-reform environment, freed from the central control and focus of the Auckland Area Health Board, South Auckland Health had a chance for a new start — but it still faced significant challenges. There are few communities in New Zealand that share the diversity of ethnicity, socioeconomic status, high child population and poor health status of the Counties Manukau region served by South Auckland Health.

There are also few communities in New Zealand that inherited public-health facilities so old and of so low a standard. The origin of its Middlemore Hospital was as a temporary facility to tend to the needs of wounded service personnel in the Second World War; those temporary facilities still form part of Middlemore Hospital.

To compound these demographic and facility problems, South Auckland Health commenced in the new health environment with a crippling operating deficit of $936,000 (NZ) on a total income of only $1.73 million.

Issues relating to health services have always existed, and this has caused many people to be negative about health reform. The reality is that the reforms as initially planned have not been implemented. What was initially planned and intended, and what has been implemented, is quite different. Apart from the critical decision not to define core health services, the reality is that monopoly purchasers are engaged in the purchase of health services from largely monopoly providers on a fundamentally historic basis.

In the absence of a "market," issues of price and performance remain to be resolved.

There are also those who deliberately wish to link the health reforms to the notion that the public-health system is likely to be privatized. In my view this will never occur, nor should it.

I have no doubt many private providers are attracted to the many low-risk aspects of health care, but I doubt many would be willing to take on the responsibility for the more complex, high-risk and costly requirements of total health services.

I believe we will always have state participation in the major provision of public-health services and the state's move to introduce normal commercial disciplines to the management of health services is quite sensible. For the first time, information systems enabling South Auckland Health to properly manage its assets, liabilities, and clinical services were being established, and services clearly defined and priced. Quality issues are being addressed. For the first time the state now knows what volume of health services it is buying when it allocates funds for the health budget.

One of South Auckland Health's intriguing new initiatives was a SuperClinic, opened in fall of 1997:

> . . . to provide a wide range of outpatient, daypatient, and day surgical services in a state of the art facility — the most sophisticated ambulatory care centre of this type in the Southern Hemisphere. It is supported by a Satellite SuperClinic at Botany Downs in Howick, where South Auckland Health is colocating with a large group of general practitioners in the same facility. The objective of colocation is to improve integration opportunities between primary and secondary sectors, with the goal of improving clinical outcomes for patients. Additional Satellite SuperClinics will be developed in other key locations.
>
> . . . The SuperClinic solution is potentially an innovative solution to many challenges, including altering demographics, increasing patient expectations, persistent downward pressure on expenditure, pressure to shift resources away from hospital-based

acute care, continued medico-technical innovation and a widespread belief that the public sector is inefficient.

Mr. Levy describes another South Auckland Health innovation in the ambulatory care area:

> While the consequences of the SuperClinic idea are highly visible, another innovative idea which has consequences that are almost invisible but its impact on clinical outcomes and altering the quality of health care is also equally significant. This progressive and innovative idea, conceived by South Auckland Health's Child Health Team, is the acute assessment of sick children at Middlemore Hospital's new Acute Assessment Unit. This assessment is undertaken by a high-powered pediatric health-care team led by a senior pediatrician. Almost two-thirds of the patients assessed are referred back home with a treatment plan as well as arranged follow-up in the home by highly trained ambulatory-care pediatric nurses. This follow-up in the home is for up to seventy-two hours and is completed by the patient being re-linked to their general practitioner. This new initiative, a first for New Zealand, has already resulted in improved clinical outcomes and a reduced number of readmissions.
>
> Innovative and constructive health-delivery solutions such as these will enhance the health status of our patients well into the new millennium. However, they may not be replaced elsewhere and may not be followed by further innovative health-delivery solutions at South Auckland Health, unless the government creates a funding/purchasing environment with appropriate and positive incentives. This will require, as a start, the elimination of Crown health enterprise deficit funding.

Lessons from South Auckland Health

Lewis Levy's hopes for South Auckland were dashed when the New

Zealand government changed. The reforms that had led to the Crown health enterprises were reversed. Yet there are at least two lessons to be learned. The first is that innovative integrated health solutions will arise regardless of nation if a larger delivery structure is created. The second is that extreme models of finance and rapid change invite controversy and reversal.

Conclusions

The movement to larger, more integrated health services–delivery organizations is evident in Sydney, Auckland, and Melbourne. The same forces of changing public expectation, financial pressures, new technologies and a broader view of health are clearly driving change in Australia and New Zealand. The Australian situation has a complexity resembling Canada's in its interplay of national and state governments; both levels of government need to be involved if change is to be achieved. New Zealand is closer to the United Kingdom in its government structures.

The reform of the U.K. National Health Service, however, pales in comparison to the degree of change undertaken in the volatile political climate of New Zealand.

14

•

Reforming the U.K. National Health Service

> ... *Britain is not alone in facing a health crisis; every Western country each year brings new and better treatments for populations that are living longer than ever. This is the insatiable demand that politicians have been citing to excuse their refusal to fund more money. But in fact there are many ways of skinning the cat.*
> — EDITORIAL, *THE BRITISH MEDICAL JOURNAL* (1998)

Margaret Thatcher had more success in implementing her vision of health-care reform in the early late 1980s than did Bill Clinton a few years later. In reshaping the National Health Service (NHS) of the United Kingdom, Prime Minister Thatcher achieved a radical reform. As discussed in Chapter 6, the changes instigated by her government caused a substantial shift of power from specialists to family doctors. They also shook up the entrenched hospital system, through the creation of trust hospitals with independent boards. These changes, while not readily embraced by either patients or providers, have survived two subsequent prime ministers, which is evidence that they were, ultimately, consistent with British values. The British reforms also preserved the confidence of the public in the NHS, making it more responsive to patients.

Another element of the British reforms was the introduction of the Patient Charter. This commitment set out what the public had a right to expect from the NHS in terms of both services and performance.

About the NHS

Unlike the fragmented Canadian health-care system, which has historically been a system for financing but not for delivering care, the United Kingdom's National Health Service is a nationwide, organized health system that strives to apply uniform standards of service and coverage. Overall responsibility for the NHS lies with the secretary of state, a member of the Cabinet. With the support of the Department of Health in London, the secretary of state develops the strategic direction for the NHS and answers to Parliament. Funding for health services is based on a weighted per capita formula under which local health authorities and GP fundholders purchase services for a population from providers such as hospitals, community services, physicians, and ambulance services.

The stated goal of the NHS is to secure the greatest possible improvement in the physical and mental health of the people of England with the resources available, by "promoting health; preventing ill health; diagnosing and treating injury and disease; and caring for those with long-term illness and disability who require the services of the NHS" (from the Department of Health's *Guide to the National Health Service*, 1996).

Established in 1948 through the leadership of Health secretary Nye Bevan, the NHS now has a budget of close to £40 billion ($96 billion

CDN) and employs nearly 1,000,000 people including employees, nurses, orderlies, and others within NHS hospitals. This makes it Europe's single largest employer.

The NHS is structured around 406 NHS "trusts" — hospitals, community service agencies, and some general practitioners. These trusts are accountable to the regional health authorities, which contract them for specific services. This division of roles between purchasers (health authorities) and providers (trusts) was a policy shift implemented under the Thatcher government in the early 1990s. The new policy was intended to increase the overall operating efficiency of the NHS by introducing some quasi-market pressures on the health care–delivery system. In theory, the health authorities became the agents of the government in identifying the health needs of the defined population, then procured the necessary services from the various trusts. Direct incentives were created for the trusts to significantly reduce their costs and provide enhanced services in order to maintain their market share.

Almost all British hospitals are self-governing NHS trusts, with the freedom to decide on staff numbers and rates of pay. The trusts are independent of the local health authority. However, they are part of the NHS and report directly to the secretary of state. Board chairs for the health authorities and NHS trusts are appointed by the secretary of state, and community health councils (which consist mainly of special-interest groups) are established in each region. Regular audits of whether the government has obtained the "best value for taxpayers' money" are also conducted by an audit commission and reported to the Public Accounts Committee.

The U.K. health-insurance scheme includes coverage for the services of physicians, opticians, dentists, health visitors (for newborns and children under five), midwives, community nurses, hospital services, physiotherapists, and occupational and speech therapists, as well as comprehensive drug benefits.

The role of general practitioners in the United Kingdom is dual in nature, in that they can act as both purchasers — through fundholding — and as providers of care. All hospital-based consultants (i.e., specialist physicians) are salaried employees of a trust. There is also a private tier of care in the United Kingdom, which provides about 15% of the country's health services.

For the most part, Britain has an integrated system of care, and hospital inpatient visits are almost always coupled with some sort of home-based care that is managed by community NHS trusts. This includes twenty-four-hour nursing/aid support and physician home visits, where required.

While the NHS costs considerably less than the Canadian system (about 6% versus nearly 10% of GNP), its economies often come at the expense of other fundamentals, such as timely access to acute-care services. There are increasing concerns among the population, providers, and policy makers about the sustainability of this approach in the foreseeable future.

As soon as the Labour government that succeeded the Thatcher Conservatives was elected, it called for a full review of the purchasing model with the intent of reducing inequities of access. The new government's first steps were to replace more than half the board chairs for the NHS trusts, to open these board meetings to the public, and to create an enhanced role for primary-care physicians in future decision making. It is too early to determine the exact implications of these changes, but they signal a significant shift toward a more populist policy agenda, and a swing away from the Thatcher era's closed, hierarchical, centrally managed approach.

As for public opinion, the NHS, while bewildering to many from other nations, remains popular at home. A survey conducted by the Commonwealth Fund, an American philanthropic organization engaged in research on health and social policy, reached the following conclusions:

As the British National Health Service (NHS) celebrates its fiftieth year, the public is happier than any other we surveyed. Amid cutbacks in other nations, the British government, which has traditionally spent far less than other nations have, has promised increases in NHS spending. Although the public notes, as it has for a decade, that the system is underfunded and waiting times for non-emergency surgery are long, Britons are least likely to call for rebuilding their health-care system and are among the least likely to be worried about future health-care needs. Britons do express some concerns about the quality of physician care. Whether this support will continue, as Prime Minister Tony Blair's honeymoon with the public fades and new reforms are undertaken, is an open question. In the meantime, there have been few changes to cause either reductions in service or increases in personal costs to patients and families. Even with reforms introduced over the past decade, the NHS has remained intact, and the result is apparently a stability of public perceptions.

— The Commonwealth Fund (1999)

Lessons from the NHS Reform

One of the driving forces behind the establishment of health authorities in the United Kingdom was the desire to make the NHS less bureaucratic in nature, and to decentralize decision making. Unfortunately, however, this has not yet fully occurred. Strong central control is actively maintained, as evidenced by the role of the state in the selection and appointment of the chairs of NHS trust and health authority boards. This creates significant tension between the national standards of service delivery and the role of the local health authorities when allocating health-care resources within their jurisdictions. The local authorities do not have the latitude to deliver a different package of health services. To achieve benefits from devolution, Canada or other nations with publicly financed health systems must be sure to *follow through* on devolution plans thoroughly, and limit central involvement in decision making.

This is easier in theory than in practice. In parliamentary democracies, the doctrine of ministerial responsibility is a force toward recentralizing. Each question a minister of health must answer with the statement that that issue is within the responsibility of the local authority tends to weaken him or her in the public view. In Alberta, the provincial government, dissatisfied with the performance of the large Calgary Regional Health Authority, fired the entire board in 1999.

The benefits of extensive integration provide a positive example for Canada and other Commonwealth countries; on the other hand, it is important to realize that the United Kingdom has spent decades developing networks of community-support services and primary care. Patient information is shared between acute and community NHS trusts, and follow-up is included as part of every patient's treatment plan. Clearly, these characteristics are fundamental to a successful integrated system.

The legacy of population-based funding has turned out to be more mixed. Although many organizations in Canada have recently begun lobbying intensely for the creation of population-based funding models, many British hospitals have learned the hard way that this model of funding does not create a stable revenue source — nor does it necessarily resolve all historical funding inequities. The purchaser/provider split has, in fact, created intense competition for survival among the 406 trusts. In response, many hospitals have developed referral management programs to ensure that patients continue to select their local-area hospital over its competitors. Canadian proponents of population-based funding schemes should note, therefore, that although this funding model may allow for revenue to be proportional to local populations, the results of fierce competition among health providers for access to the surrounding populations should not be underestimated. Canada's much larger size and sparser population may diminish the level of competition.

The NHS has found that competition among care providers on fiscal grounds yields short-term improvements in operating efficiency. However, it has also led to greater fragmentation of services as groups realign and polarization increases. Therefore, in the medium and longer term, policy makers may be faced with an even greater challenge when it comes to improving access to and coordination of care delivery. If the current "new Labour" government under Tony Blair continues the trend toward ratcheting down the funding base through direct competition, it may inadvertently erode the efficiency gains achieved to date by creating a popular backlash. This kind of reaction has its roots in a perception that efficiency has displaced access among the priorities of the NHS.

The table to the right compares the Canadian and British health systems in several major areas.

Hospital Consolidation in the United Kingdom

Despite the relative stability of the structure of the NHS, there have been significant reforms implemented, including, as in other major industrial centres, the phenomenon of hospital consolidation in London. The process has been controversial and combative; as elsewhere, great battles have been waged by supporters of hospitals slated for closure. One of the most significant, which resulted in a policy reversal in 1999, is the case of the 875-year-old St. Bartholomew's Hospital.

Plans to close St. Bartholomew's Hospital in London were reversed following a review of hospital provision in London, the Health Secretary, Frank Dobson, told MPs in the House of Commons.

"I will not countenance the closure of that great hospital, which has faithfully served the people of London for 875 years," Mr. Dobson said. . . .

Bart's will continue in its current role while the new Royal London Hospital is being built and the reorganization of other services is carried out in the east end of London. The hospital will then concentrate on its cancer and cardiac services.

Mr. Dobson said the government had accepted all the recommendations of the Turnberg review of London hospital services, which recommended that St. Bartholomew's should remain open. . . .

The recommended closure of the accident and emergency unit at Guy's Hospital will also go ahead but the situation will continue to be closely monitored. The minister's statement follows a moratorium on planned hospital closures since the general election and an

United Kingdom and Canadian Health Systems Compared

Category	United Kingdom	Canada
Jurisdiction	national system with regional implementation	provincial system with national policy framework
Funding	purchaser/provider split (incl. GP fundholding)	global funding, provincial transfer payments
Coverage	comprehensive: increasing pressure on acute-care hospital-based services	hospital inpatient and outpatient medical services, public health
Governance	state-appointed board chair for trust and health authority	independent community-based board of directors
Accountability	board of directors, NHS executive, secretary of state and audit commission	board of directors, provincial legislation corporations act
Private/Public Mix	15% private (easier access to tertiary hospital services)	28% private funds (extended insurance coverage for prescriptions, optical, semi-private, private, rehab, etc.)
General Practitioners	independent practitioners (may be fundholders)	independent practitioners
Community Support	highly developed and well integrated with hospital care	independent and often uncoordinated; moving toward integrated system
Primary Care	24-hour nursing and physician support	less developed; moving toward integrated system

Source: Zenita Hirji and Andrew Holt, "Hospitals in the U.K. Health System," *Hospital Quarterly*, Fall 1997.

independent review of the capital's health-care services by a panel chaired by Sir Leslie Turnberg, a former president of the Royal College of Physicians.

Accepting the panel's recommendations, the Health Secretary noted, "Many are in line with our proposals in the new NHS White Paper for a ten-year general improvement programme to make the NHS modern and dependable."

The report noted that in many parts of London, primary care, mental health, intermediate care, and community services were not up to standard. Mr. Dobson said an extra £140 million would be pumped into these services during the lifetime of the current Parliament.

He announced new arrangements to ensure a "London-wide strategy for health" through a regional NHS office, saying that without this, improvements would be hard, if not impossible, to achieve.

He also agreed with the panel's finding that London did not have too many acute hospital beds as presumed by the previous Conservative government.

John Maples, for the Conservatives, criticized the decision to save Bart's, saying it had not been saved for the people of east London. "Bart's will not be providing any of the local services normally provided by a district general hospital," he said.

Don Magnus of the "Save Bart's" Patient Campaign said the Accident and Emergency Department of the hospital should remain open even after East End hospital services had been reorganized, and that the fight to achieve this would continue.

While St. Bartholomew's will remain, other hospitals have been consolidated as in other countries, resulting in fewer, larger enterprises.

The University College London Hospitals' NHS Trust

University College London Hospitals' NHS trust is an example of an emergent U.K. multi-site hospital system. It comprises six hospitals at the forefront of medicine in the United Kingdom:

◇ the National Hospital for Neurology and Neurosurgery;
◇ the Middlesex Hospital;
◇ the Hospital for Tropical Diseases;
◇ the Elizabeth Garrett Anderson Hospital and the Hospital for Women, Soho;
◇ the Eastman Dental Hospital; and
◇ the University College Hospital.

University College London Hospitals is closely associated with the full-faculty University College London. Its medical school, which is closely affiliated with the hospitals, is one of the highest rated in the country.

University College London Hospitals currently operates 914 inpatient beds on its six sites. During 1996/97, it provided NHS clinical-health services to 57,823 inpatients and day cases, and provided consultations in-clinic during 380,671 outpatient attendances. The system employs more than 300 consultant medical and dental staff and 5,245 total staff, and had an income for 1997/98 of just under £203 million.

During 1997/98, University College London Hospitals delivered services to the residents of fifty-four district health authorities around the country under contract agreements made with those authorities, as well as to residents from practically every other district in the United Kingdom on a cost-per-individual-case basis. This reflects the very specialized nature of the treatment and care this trust offers.

In addition, the trust has contracts with fourteen GP fundholder practices, and with the Hackney Total Care Project — and accepts referrals from hundreds of other fundholding practices on a cost-per-individual-case basis.

Over the last three years, University College London Hospitals has worked to achieve a balanced financial plan year on year. This is not easy in a climate of change; outer London District Health Authorities wish to see as many of their patients as possible treated near their own homes in their local hospitals, reducing their dependence on some of their non-specialist services. As in other cities, the pull of services to the suburban population is very strong in London. This is the previously discussed impact of competition at work.

Conclusions

The winds of change have not spared the United Kingdom's venerable National Health Service from wrenching change. A more demanding public critical of waiting times and the unresponsive nature of health services galvanized successive governments to action. These actions have not solved all of the problems experienced by the public. They have, however, vastly increased efficiencies. The Patient Charter and an increase in the influence of family doctors are both responses to new public expectations discussed in Chapter 2. Mediated through the political system, these public demands are the most powerful driver of change in the prized but politically contentious NHS.

As well, the emergence of a broader view of health, one of the new ideas being blown in on the winds of change, motivated the development of health goals for the nation. In 1997, the newly elected Blair government appointed the first-ever U.K. Minister of Public Health. A review of inequalities in health, led by Sir Donald Acheson, was also ordered.

The financial pressures that squeezed the growth of NHS funding in the late 1980s and early 1990s sparked a consolidation of acute-care hospitals. Mergers and closures similar to those experienced in North America also characterized the U.K. hospital sector, changing delivery location for care services in that nation significantly.

At a conference I attended in the mid-1990s, Sir Duncan Nichol, a former head of the NHS, summed up the challenges facing his health system at the end of the century with the following phrases: "Case management for individuals; disease-state management for populations." They make an excellent summary of the agenda not only of the NHS but for health systems all over the developed world.

Common Themes,
Similar Challenges

Whatthings new
and different?

Regardless of whether right-leaning governments or cost-conscious
employers have driven their creation, these emergent systems have
remarkably similar characteristics.

- ⋄ Each of the systems has broadened its objectives to include the health
  of the *community* served.
- ⋄ All of the systems studied have focused on integrating their information technology and making investments in better-quality data.
- ⋄ All of the systems examined have moved to outsource the supply of
  non-clinical services, resulting often in job losses and layoffs.

◇ All of the systems have sought to integrate distinct clinical elements into a more comprehensive continuum of care.
◇ All of the systems have moved to extend the continuum of care beyond the hospital into the community and the home.
◇ The driving force in each case was a balancing of financial necessity and the desire to improve clinical performance.

As North America consolidates from the nearly 10,000 individual hospitals of its heyday into perhaps 2,000 to 3,000 health systems, a number of fascinating possibilities exist. We may move far closer to knowing how much the health of a particular population can be improved, and what are the best techniques for accomplishing this improvement. We may also learn something about efficiencies of scale: how many people can be effectively looked after by a single system? As well, we may learn about competition in health care. Can competition be used to produce better outcomes, rather than inevitably leading to the shedding of risk and inadequate coverage for some individuals? Can competition be an important tool in those countries such as Canada, the United Kingdom, Australia, and New Zealand, where the public sector bears the financial responsibility, and can it be a means for lessening the financial burden while improving the quality of care? The early results are promising but far from decisive. Cost savings are more evident in these early stages than are improvements in the quality of care, although there is some evidence of these, too.

Harder to answer are questions about what is the best way to organize the system. Is it better top-down or bottom-up? Or is that really a moot point in view of the different histories? How soon will it be before we see published a guidebook to the great health systems of the world — and which systems will it include?

Certainly we are in the midst of a major shift from a world of hospitals to a world of health systems. This convergence is evident across nations.

PART IV •

Health in the Twenty-First Century

15

•

The Health Consumer

Canadians do not want to simply be told things will be fine. They want to see it for themselves. And when they ask for information, they deserve more than ritual rhetoric; they should get a real report card.

— The Honourable Allan Rock, Minister of Health,
Speech to Canadian Medical Association (1998)

In 1993, in his Harveian Oration to the Royal College of Physicians, the distinguished British physician Sir Colin Dollery speculated about the emerging role of the consumer in health-care systems. In a teasing finale to his address, he asked whether drugs actually needed doctors. Would the pharmaceutical revolution bypass the physician and take drugs direct to patients? As noted in Chapter 8, six years after these comments, this change is in fact well under way.

This is only one of a host of ways in which the consumer is becoming a driving factor in today's health-care systems. In Chapter 1 I discussed consumerism as one of the important new ideas sweeping the sector, and in Chapter 2 I outlined, in a general sense, the changing expectations of these patient/consumers for such things as speed, quality, and appropriateness of care. This chapter presents some more detailed, concrete examples of how the notion of patients as consumers is affecting health care.

The Consumer as Care Integrator

The reality of modern health systems is that, most often, *only* the patient has an integrated view of his or her care. Many patients with chronic conditions are asked so frequently for their personal medical histories that they hand doctors a word-processed, photocopied summary.

Integration has many meanings. In the health-financing system, it refers to one-stop shopping: a single buyer of all the health services for a defined population. Integration for an American HMO is the ability to push the full risk onto provider organizations.

But integration as a concept that can fundamentally transform health services has the patient/consumer at its heart. Any vision of care integration that ignores the patient, or treats him or her as a passive participant, is sterile and will not work. Tracking patients with the precision of FedEx tracking packages but without their active involvement misses the enormous potential of the empowered patient. Unlike courier packages, patients have brains and the ability to make choices as they move along.

The chart to the right is an effort to present new models for primary care, making patients key integrators of their own care.

Primary-Care Models of Integration at Point of Care

Self-Care, Prevention, and Early Intervention

- Wellness through lifestyle changes
- Use of home self-care guide and phone care to handle most common complaints
- Informed participation with the physician in diagnosis and treatment
- Family support for chronic care

Specialty into Primary and Vice Versa

- More specialty care will be delivered in a primary-care setting
- More specialists will provide primary care for their chronically ill patients
- More "one-stop shopping" for the patient/member at convenient network-care sites

The Health Care Team

- Patient/member cared for by team of providers, not just MD
- Rigorous adherence to practice and referral guidelines
- The lowest-cost, appropriate provider sees the patient/member
- Measured according to outcomes, cost, and productivity

The "Electronic Black Bag"

- Electronic medical record
- Electronic ordering of tests, drugs, etc.
- Automated receipt of results
- Practice and referral guidelines on-line

Phone Care

- Skilled RNs handle up to 10% of today's facility encounters by phone
- RNs supported by electronic medical records, on-line triage protocols, and appointment guidelines
- A service option for members who prefer the convenience of phone care
- RNs capture assessment data for use by primary-care personnel if a hospital visit is required
- Drug and treatment compliance monitoring

The Informed Consumer

An empowered patient is an informed patient. So how does a patient become informed? The following table shows the results of a poll asking health-care consumers where they get information about health.

Sources of Consumer Health Information

Source	%
Health-Care Providers	
doctors	77
pharmacists	49
nurses	22
Other Sources	
newspapers/magazines	39
TV/radio	21
Internet	17
libraries	13

Source: Angus Reid poll, 1998.

The most dramatic change in the role of the consumer — the fact that an *informed* patient is becoming the norm — is being driven in part by the Internet revolution. For several centuries, doctors and nurses were the ones who held health information. Patients were informed on a need-to-know basis — and many health professionals had an extremely limited view of what the patient needed to know. The Internet is changing this relationship in a fundamental fashion. More than 20,000 Web sites devoted to health now provide a flood of consumer information. No longer are patients and their families dependent on the generosity of providers for information.

To illustrate the breadth, depth, and range of information available to consumers, I present just a few examples of notable health-related Web sites:

◇ InteliHealth (www.intelihealth.com) — Johns Hopkins University and Health System;

◇ HerbMed — research on 47 different herbs with links to relevant clinical studies;

◇ AmericasDoctor.com — 110 Web-connected doctors, mostly in primary care, to answer questions; and

◇ drkoop.com (www.drkoop.com) — a wide range of health-care information.

Each of these sites takes a different approach to informing the consumer. Note also the variety of ways consumers are given to judge a site's information as credible. In some cases, the reputation of an institution (such as Johns Hopkins) provides quality assurance. In others, it is an individual whose personal integrity supports the consumer's faith in the Web-based information (as in the case of former U.S. surgeon general Dr. Everett Koop). In still other cases, links are provided to scientific studies to instill consumer confidence.

The last of these sites is one of the largest health sites on the Internet, and merits a closer look.

drkoop.com: A Full-Service Health-Care Destination

Dr. C. Everett Koop is one of the most recognized names in U.S. health care. A former surgeon general, Dr. Koop enjoyed respect and a national profile in that position. The company drkoop.com has an exclusive five-year agreement (1999–2004) to license Dr. Koop's name, image, and likeness in exchange for royalty fees. Dr. Koop also serves as the company's chair.

Dr. Koop's relationship with drkoop.com created instant brand recognition and led to high Internet traffic from its inception. It also provides the company with significant influence and credibility in the market. As distrust of managed care and lack of access to physicians grows in the current, disoriented state of U.S. health care, consumers are increasingly looking for trusted sources to provide them with health-care information. On the Web, they can access information that was previously tightly controlled; they can communicate and gather insights from others with similar medical experiences and interests; and ultimately, they can gain more control of their care. Some 30 million Internet users are expected to search for health information on the Web in the year 2000.

It is drkoop.com's mission to become the most trusted consumer destination on the Internet for all health-related needs. The company seeks to accomplish this goal by providing high-quality, personalized content, services, and commerce, and by driving brand awareness and traffic through partnerships with network partners both on-line and off-line.

Whether drkoop.com will succeed in this ambitious goal remains to be seen. What is striking is the enormous pull of a well-regarded name amidst the myriad of health sites on the Internet.

Providence Health System:
The Call Centre as Patient Access Point

Although their influence is growing exponentially, Web sites are not yet the major means of supporting consumer-health relationships in the reordered health-delivery world; to date, call centres are still more prevalent in this role.

The following case study, excerpted from a paper by James Cramer and Miriam Odermann on "Patient Education Using Technology to Partner with the Consumer," provides an example of a call centre as a crucial consumer support in today's health-care environment.

> Providence Health System of Oregon has the challenge of providing consistent access to health-care services for all customers at all points of care — including four hospitals, more than twenty clinics, a number of affiliated group practices and health services, and an Oregon-wide home health service. That challenge extends to its managed care-insurance plan, Providence Health Plan, which provides insurance services to more than 190,000 plan members in

Oregon. One way Providence Health Plan is meeting its challenge is by providing access to health-care services and patient education via a medical call centre. Providence Health Plan's Care-Management Call Center strives to promote better health through education. The call center consists of four integrated services that are based on technologies and software provided by HBO & Company of Atlanta, Georgia:

— RN — The heart of Providence Health Plan's Care-Management Call Center, Providence RN is staffed by licensed nurses twenty-four hours a day, seven days a week, to provide on-line triage and medical advice to plan members only. Providence RN also outsources its services to provide after-hours coverage for community hospitals throughout Oregon. On the disease-management side of the business, in August 1998 Providence RN nurses will begin to place outbound calls to high-risk asthma patients enrolled in Providence Health Plan to ensure they are following their care plans. And call-centre nurses already use information collected in their database to make outbound calls twenty-four hours after a plan member has visited the emergency room to ensure the patient is following doctor's orders. This tactic can prevent a patient's illness from escalating to a crisis, and thereby reduces costly care encounters.

— Providence AudioLibrary — As an audiotext health information line, Providence AudioLibrary features prerecorded information, accessible by the phone, on more than 1,000 health topics, such as cardiovascular health, exercise and fitness, nutrition, smoking, and stress. Health topics are arranged in 29 categories ranging from aging to women's health issues. The information, which is available to Providence Health Plan members as well as the general population in Portland and surrounding areas, is intended to supplement information health-care consumers receive from their regular health-care providers.

— Providence Resource Line — Staffed by resource specialists,

Providence Resource Line provides services for the community as well as plan members. Sixty-five percent of the resource line's business is provider selection services. The line also refers callers to services and programs offered by Providence Health System and the community, and provides registration for health and fitness classes.

— Care Management Line — A service for physicians, the Care Management Line takes calls from primary care physicians and other health-care providers within Providence Health System that need a care manager for one of their patients or want to arrange for special health-care services, such as skilled nursing for patients with complex needs.

Because these services are integrated, at any time during a call encounter a Providence RN nurse can direct the caller to the Providence AudioLibrary to listen to automated information about the health topic he or she is interested in. Or the nurse may direct the caller to the Providence Resource Line, where a resource specialist will register the caller for a health education class. If the consumer first calls in to the Providence Resource Line, he or she may also be directed to the Providence AudioLibrary, and so forth. Further integration is planned between the call centre and the electronic medical record (EMR) so that call encounters will be entered into the patient's permanent medical record and nurses can access the patient's medical history.

Finally, in fall 1998, Providence Health System's information-services department will embark on a pilot project in which the medical call centre will be the integrator of all information systems, including the core hospital information system, the electronic medical record, and the health-plan database. By putting the medical call centre in the middle of the health-enterprise model, it becomes a consumer's point of entry into the health system. This will enable Providence to meet its vision of providing consistent access to health-care services by directing the health-care consumer to the right place and the right information in one phone call.

Providence Health Plan's Care-Management Call Center has been well received by plan members. In fact, customer satisfaction with the plan overall led to a four-star rating in 1997 and 1998 by *U.S. News and World Report*, which gave the top honor to just thirty-seven health plans nationwide. While the call centre can't accept all the credit, it was a key contributor in maintaining customer satisfaction and loyalty to the plan. More concrete results can be found in the yearly surveys Providence Health Plan conducts of its plan members. The most recent study (conducted in 1997) shows that 20% of the plan's 193,000 members call Providence RN each year for medical advice, accounting for the call centre's 3,100 calls per month. (These numbers do not include calls into the Providence AudioLibrary and Providence Resource Line by members of the community seeking general health information.) Of the plan members who have placed a call to Providence RN, callers rated the nurses' helpfulness to them 4.28 on a scale of 1 to 5, with 5 meaning excellent. Callers also said the advice was easy to understand, giving that category a rating of 4.42, and overall service received a 4.49. Perhaps the most telling statistic is that 46.7% of the callers were able to care for themselves at home as a result of advice given to them by a Providence RN nurse. This means that a significant number of people each month avoided costly visits to the emergency room or even to their primary-care physicians.

The Providence Health System is an example of the hundreds of health systems that are using call centres to separate information delivery from the patient visit, as discussed in this chapter.

Health Guides and Report Cards

Another tool that is helping the growing consumer-support role of health care is the health guide, or report card. These guides and ratings are a way of letting consumer/patients have some insight into what to expect and where to expect it before entering the health-care system at a particular point. As the *Journal of the American Medical Association* commented in 1997, "Consumer reports are gaining a great deal of attention from consumer groups, health-care delivery organizations such as hospitals and managed care organizations, and physicians. They are included as a requirement in many state and national health-care reform proposals. . . . By facilitating clinician and provider organization accountability and informing consumers, consumer guides may improve health-care quality and reduce costs."

A health guide answers questions such as the following: How do I navigate my local health system? How do I get the care I need? Where should I go with my condition? These questions are basic, but right now the answers to them are not always apparent to the public.

A report card measures health care in a statistical way: How long is it going to take me to get access, and what are the waiting times? What's the quality of the service that I'm going to get? Are the outcomes for this treatment better at this hospital than at that hospital, or in this city than that other city? How quickly can I expect to be treated? Will I get the most appropriate care based on my health needs and the best scientific evidence?

Measuring health-care outcomes is definitely not a new idea; Florence Nightingale lamented the lack of information on health services and their effectiveness a century ago. Although formal health-care report cards for organizations are new to Canada, they have been used elsewhere — in the United States and Great Britain — with success. In some U.S. states, hospitals are mandated by law to provide report cards that include such information as how well their health-care providers are performing surgeries, what the complication rates are for certain treatments, and how often patients are readmitted to hospital after treatment.

The "league tables" published in England, Scotland, and Wales are a form of report card. Hospitals there are rated with one to five stars in fifty-nine areas according to how well they meet their targets in treating patients. For example, patients are supposed to be seen by a triage nurse within five minutes of arriving in an emergency ward, with the exception of trauma victims or other seriously injured or sick people, who are whisked in and put under a doctor's care right away. Hospitals that rank less than three out of five stars have some explaining to do at the board and community level.

Measuring time targets is one way a jurisdiction can ease into report cards before moving on to more controversial aspects of measuring care, such as the rate of complications and even deaths. The purpose of publishing this kind of ranking is to bring public pressure to bear for improved performance into the hospital and health system.

A number of U.S. states have become very involved in health-care quality measures. New York State publishes a consumer guide. Missouri has a terrific guide to its hospitals. It's very simple: you look up the hospital that you're supposed to go to and it tells you that, for example, in delivering a baby this hospital does better than average, average, or worse than average. For heart surgery and a number of serious procedures, the ranking can help a patient be comfortable — "I'm going to a place that's above average" — or mildly comfortable — "They're average" — or a little worried — "Maybe this isn't the best place to go; maybe I should ask my doctor about alternatives."

Although report cards were rarely mentioned in health-care discussions a couple of years back, they are rapidly becoming very popular in Canada. The Ontario Hospital Association has already published a report on the hospital system, and in 1998 and 1999 they published the rates of surgical and medical complications for various procedures by hospital name, as well as readmission rates, patients' satisfaction with health care, and even information on hospital finances. Some Toronto teaching hospitals have also published their own report cards. And the federal and provincial governments, recognizing the need for accountability within the new "social union" framework agreed to by nine provinces, will begin in the next four years to report on health and social outcome measures.

One problem with reporting results in Canada is that the report cards being developed up to now, while laudable, are voluntary. Any hospital that does not want to participate in the Ontario Hospital Association's report card doesn't have to. Perhaps Canada will follow the lead of several American states and mandate report cards by law. That way, hospitals and doctors would have to provide information on death and complication rates in a uniform manner. Patients would be assured of comparable data from all hospital sites.

Of course, just putting out the information alone isn't always the answer. An objective watchdog body to make sure hospitals meet at least minimum standards is necessary, so patients don't become victims of medical malpractice or poor hospital management.

Several Canadian organizations, such as the Institute for Clinical Evaluative Sciences and the Manitoba Centre for Health Policy and Evaluation, have done good work, but they've tended to focus on either how to make better government policy or on how patient-care decisions are made by providers. The first of these organizations is based in Ontario and has an emphasis on clinical epidemiology — the patterns of disease. The second, based in Winnipeg, uses administrative data to advise on health policy. For example, to determine whether or not hospitals are doing too many Caesarean sections, rates at different hospitals and their outcomes are compared. The "practice atlases" developed in Ontario by the Institute for Clinical Evaluative Sciences provide excellent information on patterns of care, but they are written for a readership of policy makers and practitioners, not health-care consumers.

We need to translate that work into a more user-friendly style, and add still more information that is relevant to a consumer, so that a report card actually means something to the average person. The consumer needs easy access to the answers to a range of questions, such as "How healthy am I? How healthy is my community? How do I know if I'm really sick? How do I know if my child has appendicitis? And what should I do about it? If I'm going to have a particular surgery — where's the best place to get it?"

Groups of people with specific health problems have started asking some very pointed questions about whether they're getting appropriate service. A few years ago in Ontario, the issue of breast-conserving surgery received a fair amount of attention. It became apparent that where a woman went for breast-cancer care often affected the treatment she received more than did the details of her condition. That is, some hospitals favoured radical mastectomies, while others did a lot of lumpectomies. Consumers — in this case, women with breast cancer — were indignant; they wanted to be assured of treatment that was appropriate to their health condition, regardless of where they went.

Provider organizations are usually eager to collect data for use in benchmarking so that they can manage better, but they often show real reluctance when it comes to providing too much specific information to consumers. An organization's questions differ from a consumer's.

The measurement process can also be stressful for providers. The reality of report cards is that not everybody is going to get an A. Especially in the first round, there is a tendency to deny the results — "there must be something wrong with the numbers" — and an urge to "shoot the messenger." Change is at first resisted in health services, but often gradually embraced. Eventually a health-care culture develops from the feedback loop; a bad grade means simply "we had better do something to fix this." Once there is a standard in place that's clear to everyone, people want to affect it. Just as players want to improve their batting averages in the major leagues, so surgeons want to reduce their complication rates. Peer pressure also comes to bear once that data are out there and available.

Managers of the health system — at the government, hospital, or regional authority level — would love to run the system more on the basis of evidence of what's being achieved for the resources being expended; report cards are one very good tool for doing this. (For more on evidence-based health policy, see Chapter 18.) In the absence of that kind of transparency, judging organizations is often a largely political exercise, involving a great deal of passionate argument without much in the way of supporting facts.

At the very least, report cards allow patients to have true, informed consent. Every day, patients turn over their bodies to doctors and hospitals with few questions asked. In fact, most of us can find out more about how our hotels and restaurants rate than our hospitals and doctors. At the very least, patients deserve to know not only the history and risks associated with the procedure but also those associated with the pair of hands performing it.

In the United States, risk-adjusted deaths for coronary artery–bypass graft surgery have dropped dramatically. Report cards have accelerated quality improvement. Service levels have also improved, particularly for maternal care, as it has become easier for women to get information on how various institutions compare.

The drive for report cards that challenge and question hospitals, doctors, and health-care providers is really an offshoot of the larger trend toward more accountability to society on the part of various institutions: governments, political leaders, clergy — and health-care systems. Gone are the days of no questions asked. Patients and the public are far more challenging and skeptical of public institutions — and rightly so.

Conclusions

Health systems are adapting to the consumer in three important ways: more transparency through report cards; easier access through call centres and Web sites; and more support for self-care.

The report-card movement is gaining momentum. This is clear evidence of the rise of the consumer in the health-care marketplace. Whether people are seeking care in an organized, informed way, or shopping for care with a greater degree of activism, the implication for health services is clear: meet the test of transparency or face the wrath of consumers. Another clear risk is that consumers will "vote with their feet" as they seek out the most forthcoming, highest-quality service providers.

The explosion in health call centres and health Web sites is further evidence of consumers demanding more and better information. No longer are people willing to wait for the pronouncements of their doctors. Faced with symptoms or worries, they seek instant information by telephone or by computer. Health information once travelled home in the form of a doctor's verbal advice or a written prescription; in the new world of health information, it is only a telephone call or a keystroke away. And we are still in the early stages of the chip-enabled, consumer-driven revolution in health services. Faster, more comprehensive, more personalized health information is the likely next frontier.

Providing health information is an important foundation for the movement toward self-care — but it is only a beginning. The trend toward providing many medications over the counter (see Chapter 8) furthers this direction. As well, there is a proliferation of home-testing products available, from pregnancy tests to blood-pressure and glucose monitors. Particularly for those with chronic conditions, such as diabetes or heart disease, the ability to manage one's own care with more accurate, self-administered tests can enhance quality of life. The chip-driven push toward miniaturization and lower-cost diagnostic technologies will also boost self-care.

Today's health-care consumer is the more informed, more aggressive alter ego of yesterday's patient. This transformation is likely to accelerate, not slow down, in the coming years.

16

•

Managing Demand

Our contention is that, unless we address the demand side of the equation meaningfully, we will never truly cope with the challenges of a changing society's demand for a different sort of health system.

— DAVID PENCHEON, INSTITUTE OF PUBLIC HEALTH WEB SITE, CAMBRIDGE UNIVERSITY (AUGUST 1997)

In 1994 I wrote my first book, *Healing Medicare: Managing Health System Change the Canadian Way*. In the course of the research for that book, I became intrigued with the demand side of the health-care equation. Along with nearly everyone else involved in the health-care industry, the overwhelming focus of my thinking had been on the supply side: reengineering the care-delivery system. However, I did include a very short chapter entitled "Managing Demand for Health Services." Since 1994, the fledgling field of demand management has expanded, gaining both depth and controversy along the way. This comes from the impressive range of efforts that have been undertaken to reconcile demand with need. The controversy stems from a misuse of demand management as a technique for rationing or denying care to those with genuine needs.

This chapter was inspired by three sources. The first was an article by Dr. C. Everett Koop, the former U.S. surgeon general cited in the previous chapter, and a number of others, published in the *New England Journal of Medicine* in July 1993. The article, "Reducing Health-Care Costs by Reducing the Need and Demand for Medical Services," sparked my interest in the demand side of the health-care equation. It was a bold, thoughtful piece of work that attempted to bring together a great deal of the documented work on the demand side. Historically, this has not been seen as a coherent body of work, but this article broke new and important ground in shaping the way the health-care community thinks.

My second formative experience in this area was a long walk in the green but very muddy pastoral setting of Ditchley Park in Oxfordshire, England, in 1993 with Dr. Jack Wennberg. As our big rubber boots slopped in the mud, John held forth on his views. Informed patient choice and shared decision making are where Dr. Wennberg and the group that he has inspired at the Dartmouth Medical School place their emphasis. According to the philosophy of "informed patient choice," there is no one right medical answer for most patients and most medical conditions. Instead, the starting point is the view that a range of options and risks exists in any given situation, all of which the patient needs to take into account in coming to a decision about how to deal with his or her medical condition.

So how does the notion of informed patient choice inspire a chapter on demand management? Well, it stands to reason that a more informed patient will use health services more appropriately. This will mean less use in many instances — but not always. "Patients," intoned Dr. Wennberg, "are more risk averse than their surgeons." And properly so.

The third inspiration was spending six months at the Centre for

Bioethics at the University of Toronto. There I encountered Dr. Peter Singer and others who had done extensive work in developing a practical living will. This forward-thinking directive allows healthy people to determine in advance how much or how little treatment they would like in the event they ever become incapacitated. The centre's *Living Will* is a bestseller.* The kind of advanced directives it helps people create have been legislatively sanctioned in many provinces and states. Here is a tool that offers health-care consumers the ability to manage their own demand, in advance, at a high-stress, high-intervention, high-cost point in the health cycle, often toward the end of their lives.

Moving Forward

Since I wrote *Healing Medicare* in 1994, the activities directed toward managing demand have increased exponentially. Some activities have taken a negative view of the subject, associating managing demand with restricting access to care. This is unfortunate; it is impossible to completely understand the next health-care revolution without a grasp of the effects of managing demand for health services. Across North America, this revolution is taking hold as integrated health–delivery systems emerge. As care delivery consolidates and shifts to an outcome or evidence base, the need to manage both the supply of and the demand for services will grow.

Although Canada and the United States take quite different approaches to health care, certain convergences are under way (see Chapters 11 and 12). In Canada, where governments are the major single payers, they are devolving authority to regional bodies, which will rapidly become interested in managing demand for services in view of their capped budgets. In the United States, the rapid emergence of integrated-delivery networks providing care is also sparking interest in managing demand. As both providers and payers consolidate in the United States, it is clear that lives will be managed and "owned" in health-care terms for longer

---

* This document is available from the Centre for Bioethics, 88 College Street, Toronto, Ontario, M5G 1F2. Fax (416) 978-1911.

and longer periods of time. Therefore, the incentives will increase to manage those lives to optimum health, so as to defer expensive treatment costs in time or eliminate them all together.

Looking Ahead

Attention must shift from the supply side of health-care delivery to the demand side of the cost and quality equation. Across North America, a revolution in demand management is under way. Consumers, providers, and health-care managers have projected the belief that the demand for health-care services is fixed, rising, and unmanageable. If we can manage only the supply of health-care services, then we devote all our attention to half the problem. If, as many leaders believe, demand is also subject to management, then we are in the early stages of a true revolution. The work of many — be they architects of advanced directives, advocates and designers of informed patient choice, or proponents of population health — is contributing to the overturning of traditional thought and action in health care. From passively accepting the behaviour of health-care consumers and providers, policy makers are slowly moving to a new approach of informing — and, by informing, altering and managing that behaviour.

Access Health, profiled in detail in Chapter 17, is an example that has captured, in its relatively brief corporate history, this dramatic swing of the American health-care pendulum. Established initially as a nurse call-line service, Access Health marketed itself to hospitals, suggesting that such a call line could gain greater customer loyalty. More patients would visit the hospital, drawn by the friendly, accessible service.

In fact, exactly the opposite occurred. Hospitals found that when their customers had access to credible information by telephone, visits dropped dramatically. Better informed patients were able to eliminate many trips to the health-care facility on their own. Access Health quickly shifted its emphasis to the other side of the marketplace, realizing that payers, not providers, were their natural customer base, with an interest in reducing the number of visits and the volume of services provided.

What will our future health-care system look like? Across North America, some 10,000 individual hospitals will come together in integrated health–delivery networks, with perhaps fewer than 1,000 of them in operation by the early part of the twenty-first century. As these integrated networks and their payers, larger and larger health-maintenance organizations (HMOs) and regional health authorities, increasingly take total responsibility for the health of significant populations, new incentives will shift their focus. Rather than working toward efficiency in each transaction, they will begin looking across the life spectrum to see how they can provide effective quality care. At the top of the list will be keeping the consumer healthy.

Other factors discussed throughout this book will also contribute, in various ways, to an increased emphasis on keeping the demand for health services down. The pharmaceutical industry will evolve through the intermediate stage of pharmaceutical benefit management toward disease-state management (see Chapter 19). Companies will enroll people with risk factors and seek, over a period of time, to prevent them from developing cardiovascular disease or diabetes. They will also seek to manage the early stages of these diseases. The pendulum will swing still further as we all become more aware of the preventable illnesses and deaths, and greater and greater regulations come to fall upon the tobacco industry and its marketing of illness and death.

Similarly, further advances in keeping patients informed will fuel demand management. Besides call lines or the Mayo Clinic CD or health information on-line, patients will increasingly have access to pharmaceuticals over the counter. As discussed in Chapter 8, direct-to-consumer marketing by the pharmaceutical industry is increasing, sometimes going as far as full-page ads. If you know that when certain symptoms turn up and you take your child to the doctor, he or she is going to write you the same prescription for the sixteenth time, you may be inclined to think, "Maybe I could just go to the pharmacist and say, 'Here is the last prescription, fill it again.'" I know there are all sorts of arguments against this kind of scenario, but the fact is that this kind of unbundled process is going on, driven by increased consumer confidence and access to information. I think another trend you'll see is a huge movement toward patients being able to access their own records.

Conclusions

As the management of demand in health care becomes a more sophisticated activity, it will be increasingly tailored to the individual. Enabled by advances in technology, health systems will seek to reduce the use of high-cost health services in the acute-care setting. The techniques available for substituting self-care and more robust primary care for higher activity care are improving. With closer-to-home diagnostics, demand management will, I hope, shed its earlier connotations of building barriers to access while forging a true partnership between the health system and patients and their families.

17

•

Chip-Driven Companies
and "eHealth"

The http://www.com changes everything.

— ANONYMOUS SAYING INVOKED AT ALL INTERNET CONFERENCES

The notion of "eHealth" is the application of digital technology to the health-services sector — specifically, the transformation of key business, clinical, and patient-care processes using Internet/intranet technologies. Three clusters of chip-based activity in health information technology can be identified: traditional health-care information technology, such as point-of-care computing and the "wiring" of individual hospitals; health-care information networks, usually linking various providers; and, of course, the Internet/World Wide Web and the phenomenal number of health-related Web sites now available.

The convergence of Internet technology, the silicon chip, and various aspects of the health-care business is leading to a revolution, and to astonishing growth in health-related technology businesses, as shown by this review of a few leading-edge companies.

On-line Health and the Smart Investor

A May 26, 1999, report by Wit Capital, an online investment banking and brokerage firm, stated that the future of health care is "on (the) line." Four reasons were advanced:

1. The Internet has transformed the fundamental structures of many industries, from financial services to book retailing. . . . Health care is a particularly attractive industry to benefit from Web-based technologies due to its enormous size, inefficiency, and information intensity. A number of emerging, entrepreneurial eHealth companies seek to leverage the power of the Internet to improve communications, streamline workflow, and generate new revenue opportunities in health care.

2. The revenue opportunities in eHealth are enormous and include e-commerce, connectivity, and advertising/sponsorship. We estimate the scale of the e-commerce opportunity to be several hundreds of billions of dollars, the connectivity market to be several billion dollars, and the advertising opportunity to be hundreds of millions of dollars.

3. We believe that successful eHealth companies will share certain fundamental characteristics, including a first-mover advantage, differentiated products or services, a strong brand, rapidly building scale, and multiple revenue streams.

4. We note that the complex, sensitive nature of health-care information and products poses a unique set of challenges, including security and privacy, government regulation, physician adoption, and technology hurdles. We expect that those companies best able to address these issues will build significant competitive advantage over the next several years.

Wit goes on to explain that we are in the early days in the eHealth industry.

> While only a handful of companies thus far have accessed the public markets, a considerable number are waiting in the wings. Private equity capital continues to pour into this area, and a number of heavyweights, including Microsoft, Intel, Merck, Amazon.com and DuPont, have staked claims through strategic investments and partnership. . . .

Notwithstanding these issues, we believe a number of characteristics make health care a particularly attractive industry to benefit from the continued growth of the Internet, including:

- An Enormous Market — Health care is the largest sector in the U.S. economy, accounting for over $1 trillion (U.S.) in annual spending, or 14% of the GDP. We believe that a number of segments are particularly attractive, including health insurance ($500+ billion), pharmaceuticals ($100 billion in the United States; $300+ billion worldwide) and medical supplies and products ($100+ billion).
- Inefficiency — The health-care industry is notoriously inefficient. Companies woefully underinvest in technology, and business processes remain labour-intensive and largely paper-based, with significant duplication of effort.
- Information Intensity — Herein lies a dramatic irony: health care is one of the most information-intensive industries, yet it lacks the technological infrastructure necessary to capture, store, and access much of that information. It is remarkable that physicians can receive real-time financial information to manage personal portfolios but cannot access an electronic patient chart in the operating room.
- A Broad, Attractive Customer/User Base — Health care affects every person's life and consistently ranks at the top of on-line users' interests. According to CyberDialogue, over 22 million

U.S. adults search for health information on the Internet, and this number is expected to reach 30 million by 2000. Also according to CyberDialogue, these "HealthMed retrievers" are wealthier, more educated, and have more Internet experience than the average on-line user.

— Fragmentation — Health care is an industry consisting of hundreds of thousands of disparate entities: payers, hospitals, physicians, laboratories, and pharmacies, among many others. Each organization maintains legacy systems with different hardware, software, and platforms, making it extremely difficult to communicate and exchange information.

Clearly, the health sector is ripe for a transformation using digital technology.

What companies are leading the way? Wit defines four clusters of companies. The first category, which it calls "context," includes Ad.com; drkoop.com; On-Health, and Medi-consult. The second cluster, which includes the fast-growing Healtheon, is entitled "connectivity," and also includes Careinsight, and Claimsnet.com. In the eHealth/e-commerce group are drugstore.com, endsweb, quotesmith, and Camdex. And finally, in the health–information technology area, the names — familiar to many hospital managers — of Cerner, Shared Medical Services, Proxy-med, and HBOC are included. It is worth noting that these companies in some instances command quite remarkable market caps — for example, Healtheon's is $2.4 billion (U.S.); drugstore.com's, a little over $2 billion; and Careinsight's, $3.1 billion.

A few examples of companies that I believe exemplify or symbolize the future of the digitally driven health system are profiled below.

Healtheon

Healtheon was started in 1996. Its founder, the colourful Jim Clark, had also founded Netscape and Silcon Graphics, two of the most successful digital technology firms. Jim Clark's belief was that the Internet should have been used until 1996 for E-mail, publishing, and simple transactions, and afterwards to support mainstream commerce and complex mission-critical transactions. His view was that there was a unique benefit to be had from a high degree of digital integration in the health-care sector because of its size, degree of fragmentation, and importance to society.

Healtheon's mission, as described on its Web site, is "to leverage advanced Internet technology and connect all participants in health care, to enable them to communicate and exchange information and perform transactions which cut across the health-care maze." Its business model is described in simpler, cruder terms by Jim Clark: "We want to empower the doctors and the patients and get all the other assholes out of the way. Except for us. One asshole in the middle."

The first task for Healtheon was to develop a robust platform that could integrate health information. By mid-1997, Healtheon launched its first transaction between consumers and health plans, including electronic enrollment, provider selection, and health-care benefits management for a number of health insurers in the United States and in Canada. By the fall of 1997, Healtheon had entered into a relationship with Brown & Tolland, a large physician organization in northern California, to develop Internet-based services to connect physicians to health plans. More specifically, these services would manage eligibility enquiries, referrals, authorizations, claims submissions, provider directories, and information reporting. In the same year, 1997, Healtheon connected with Beech Street, the nation's largest IPO, to create Internet services to manage a provider network of 300,000 physicians, support claims, and repricing transactions. In 1997, Healtheon acquired one of the fastest-growing electronic data–interchange providers, Acta-Med Corporation.

In 1998, Healtheon acquired Metic LLC, a leading consulting and application-development firm. In 1999 came Healtheon's largest acquisition yet: WebMD, a leading health Internet site.

Healtheon is not alone in its attempts to wire the health system together using digital technology. However, the breadth of its vision and the strength of its leadership suggest that Healtheon will have a major impact on this sector. Jim Clark changed the game in the computer industry with Netscape and Silicon Graphics. As founder and chairman of Healtheon, he provides strong leadership. By late 1998, Healtheon could boast a major customer network that included 67,000 physicians, 450 payers, and some 25 million administrative electronic transactions, and a further 250 million clinical electronic transactions.

The acquisition of WebMD makes Healtheon much more of an interface between the consumer and the health-care system, and raises the profile of the firm with those consumers seeking information through the Internet.

Prior to its acquisition by Healtheon, WebMD Inc., of Atlanta, Georgia, had embarked on an ambitious campaign to overtake its rivals and establish itself as the world's premier health-care Web site. The company was well financed — it had received investments of $360 million (U.S.) from a range of companies, including Microsoft, Intel, Excite, Softbank, and Superior Consultant Co.

WebMD attracted attention when it announced its merger with Healtheon. For its part, WebMD plans to spend $265 million (U.S.) on marketing and promotion over the next five years to establish the site — and the name WebMD — as an international brand. The company will be running a massive advertising campaign to attract attention, including TV, radio, and Web banner ads.

As well as spending on advertising and promotion, WebMD has announced a flurry of significant marketing agreements and strategic moves in recent months that may help it to gain ground.

The Web site is developing into a producer of medical content, where previously it was merely an aggregator of information. Aggregators point visitors to other sites that provide information, such as publications, universities, companies, or similar organizations with Web pages. Healtheon now has plenty of its own copy to post, with seventy-five full-time writers on staff working in concert with twenty-five physicians.

Footmaxx

Not all of the chip-driven change is flowing from gigantic global firms. A myriad of much smaller firms are also applying the power of the digital revolution to old ways of doing things in health-care services. One example of this phenomenon is Footmaxx, based in Toronto, Canada.

Let me declare my conflict of interest at the outset. Lawrence & Company, where I work in the investment world, has a major stake in Footmaxx. As well, I sit on the board of directors and chair the executive committee. I do not believe, however, that making reference to it in this book is likely to cause the share price to rocket. My reason for including Footmaxx is that it is a tiny, perfect example of the phenomenon I'm trying to document. (Although it is not, I add with some pride, so tiny any more. . . .) Footmaxx is a digital-technology company with a future.

The old way of making orthotics for people's feet was to take a plaster mould of the foot, and then use that mould as the basis for building the orthotic by hand. This kind of orthotic, when inserted into a shoe, can help improve not only a foot problem but, since the foot bone is connected to the ankle bone, and eventually (as the song goes) to the knee bone and the thigh bone, the use of orthotics has an important positive impact for people with, for example, some kinds of back pain that are, ultimately, foot related.

The innovative founder of Footmaxx, Dr. Glenn Copeland, working with skilled information-technology people, developed a gait analysis based on scanning the foot for pressure points. You walk across a simple platform the size of a bathroom rug, and a number of points of pressure are measured. From this, a computer image is generated, and from that computer image an orthotic is built. No plaster, no mess — and much greater accuracy in the construction of the orthotic.

To date, Footmaxx is more of a technological triumph than a financial success, although that success will likely follow, in due course. Some 1,000 physicians across North America, largely foot specialists, have purchased Footmaxx's machines and begun using them to prescribe orthotics for their patients.

At the heart of Footmaxx, as with the other companies examined, is the silicon chip. The old plaster methodology has been replaced by three separate high-tech innovations: the chip's power to record data and allow it to be analyzed, the scanning technology, and the mat that measures the gait. Footmaxx is clearly part of the digital health revolution, albeit not on the same scale as Healtheon. But just as the digital revolution is enabling Healtheon to reengineer how health transactions are carried out, it is allowing Footmaxx to reengineer how the examination of a foot and the prescription for an orthotic are carried out.

Access Health

One of the most interesting places I had a chance to visit in the mid-1990s was a health business in Sacramento, California, called Access Health. Here I saw for the first time the future of health care on the telephone. At that time, Access Health was promoting itself as a company running nurse call lines. That is a significant understatement. One of the responses to the high cost of initial visits (especially in the United States, where it is common to see a specialist on the first visit) has been telephone information. Health insurers like Blue Cross give people in California a kit that has a sticker for the phone and a magnet for the fridge bearing a phone number and a slogan that encourages calling Access Health before rushing off to the doctor or to the emergency room.

Access hires only nurses with at least ten years of experience; almost all were trained in the emergency room or operating room. They sit in a room with computer consoles and answer the phone. Access gets a lot of repeat business; consumers have confidence that the nurses will provide them with useful and trustworthy information.

Supported by computer protocols, the nurses are very careful on the line, so as not to give out misleading information or risk misdiagnosing an illness. While I was visiting the facility I said to them, "What you're doing is primary care!" and they replied, "Oh, no, it's just an information service." But according to my observation, the service is much more than information; it is a true part of primary care.

One result of this service is that 85% of the people who were planning to go to the emergency don't go after they've had a conversation with a nurse. About 2% or 3% of them get rushed right in because they have symptoms that suggest an urgent problem; the individual is told to stay on the line, and an ambulance is called immediately. But more often a nurse will find herself speaking, for example, to an elderly woman who has just been to her weekly bridge club lunch, had a little too much to drink, and felt dizzy when she got home. A phone chat about her symptoms with the nurse reassures her that no visit to the emergency room is needed — the computer reminds both caller and nurse that this dizziness is a frequent post-bridge-club phenomenon.

The basic concept behind this info line is to unbundle the information from the visit. Rather than spending three hours coming down to the emergency room to determine whether or not he or she even needs the emergency room, a consumer can actually often solve the problem immediately, at home, with some information.

Callers also have the option of "visiting" Access's audio library, which offers information on about 600 topics. (The most commonly accessed topics are "How Do I Know if I'm Pregnant?" and "How Do I Know if I Have a Sexually Transmitted Disease?") Consumers want information; at one time the only way to get that information was to visit the doctor, but often a person would much rather just get the information. Informed health consumers, as discussed in Chapters 15 and 16, are empowered — both as consumers and as managers of their own care.

Insurers are paying for telephone health–access lines. The cost is about $8 (U.S.) a year per enrolled person. To put that amount into context, total health-care costs per person per year in Canada average about $1,800 (CDN), and in the United States about $2,800 (U.S.); Access guesses that the savings to providers average between $100 and $200 (U.S.) per enrolled person — while increasing customer satisfaction. "This Personal Health Advisor thing has raised our rating by 8 percentage points. Nothing else we've ever done has made people as happy," commented one health-plan executive. "Even customers who did not use it liked the idea that they had this kit and the phone number available twenty-four hours a day."

There are several kinds of abuse in the health-care system, and the hardest one to eliminate is not malicious abuse, but people moderately overusing the system "to be on the safe side." Some $200 million (CDN) a year is spent in Ontario with people going to the doctor with common colds. How do you solve this problem? You do not want to miss the symptoms that are really viral pneumonia. The public is, understandably, hard to move in terms of attitude if there is no alternative to a physician visit. Reliable information available by telephone is a smart, win-win solution.

Tunstall: The Caring Network

For a fascinating example of a product that uses modern information and telecommunications technology to improve both quality and affordability, a look at the British company Tunstall PLC is worthwhile. Tunstall started out in the alarm business, and thirty years later it has evolved into a high-technology manufacturer. One of its leading-edge products is called The Caring Network. The company describes it thus:

> The Caring Network is a clever use of telecommunications technology and people to provide the elderly with security in their homes while assisting the management of in-home services.
>
> The elements of the system are straightforward: a special, modified telephone for the person's home, a control switchboard staffed by trained personnel, and a computer capable of tracking and storing an accessible record of all care provided.
>
> The Caring Network system allows elderly persons to remain in their home with the security of immediate access to care and a friendly, familiar voice by telephone. By including the record-keeping function for all home visits, the system begins to dramatically reduce the paperwork burden on providers.

Recently, Tunstall tackled the issue of accidental falls in the home. Their focus on falls had three key data points to support it.

◇ Every five hours in the United Kingdom, an older person is killed by an accidental fall in the home.
◇ Over 300,000 U.K. pensioners are so seriously injured by a fall in their home that they require hospital treatment.
◇ Hip fractures, which are the most common injury caused by falls, cost the U.K. National Health Service an estimated £160 million a year, and account for 20% of all hospital orthopedic beds. One in five who suffer a hip fracture die within six months.

Tunstall has developed a new piece of equipment, which it describes as follows:

Tunstall and the Telecare company Technology in Healthcare are designing a sensor with the ability to raise the alarm when a person has fallen. The recent launch of the Government's "Avoiding Slips, Trips and Broken Hips" campaign makes the development of a fall detector particularly timely.

The Department of Trade and Industry, in partnership with the Health Education Authority, has launched a three-year initiative to reduce the number of deaths and injuries due to falls, which are the largest single kind of accident in the home. The risk of falling increases significantly as people get older. While the fall itself may not be life-threatening, if the person lies undiscovered for any length of time, the consequences can be more severe. Future falls may then become more likely, each subsequent fall bringing an increased risk of fracture or serious injury.

The fall detector, which has been granted "Millennium Product" status by the Design Council, will provide reassurance to older, disabled, and other vulnerable people who fear being left unable to summon help following an accident or collapse in the home.

Tunstall and Technology in Healthcare are conducting trials with a number of volunteer users and care professionals. The results so far have been very encouraging. "The fall detector is the first of a range of TeleHealth devices being developed for use with community alarms," said Andrew McIntosh, Project Manager; "They have the potential to help many elderly and disabled people maintain their independence and continue living safely in their own homes."

Tunstall and others in the field are using chip-based technology to equip homes with many of the same security features as hospitals.

The Data Chip in Your Toilet Bowl

Matsushita, a major Japanese technology company, has developed a high-tech health-information toilet. Available by the end of the year 2000, this chip-based wonder will measure your body temperature, weight, and blood pressure. By 2003, Matsushita plans to add features to test the amounts of glucose and protein in urine.

A further innovation from the same company is the Vital Signs Kit, intended to improve home care. It contains everything from the old world of health care, such as a thermometer and a blood-pressure gauge, as well as features for the new wired world, such as a built-in videophone for consultations with remote physicians. A blood-sugar monitor allows readings to be sent by phone or Internet to the clinic. This technology is a further illustration of the unbundling of diagnostics and care from hospital to clinic to home. It allows the remote management of care by providers as well as a greater degree of self-care by patients.

Blue Gene

In 1997, IBM's Deep Blue Computer beat the world chess champion. Two years later, in 1998, IBM announced the launch of project "Blue Gene." Their $100 million (U.S.) plan is to build a new RS/6000 computer to help unlock the mysteries of human genetics, model proteins, and help pharma companies design drugs. Blue Gene will be 1,000 times more powerful than Deep Blue; clearly, IBM believe in the continuing validity of Moore's Law.

Design Your Own Tour

The best way to understand the full impact of the digital revolution on health care is to go for a virtual tour yourself. If your computer is not up to the task, locate the nearest child — he or she is likely to possess the computer, the bandwidth, and the skills you will need to visit some health-related Web sites and get the lay of the land.

My suggestion for a tour of the top-three health Web sites is as follows:

1. www.drkoop.com (see Chapter 15)
2. www.webmd.com (see discussion of Healtheon, above)
3. www.mayohealth.org (the Mayo Clinic's site)

Conclusions

Chip-driven, innovative companies such as the ones discussed above and thousands of others will transform the traditional landscape of health care. Understanding the key implications of these new technologies is essential to the success of these ventures in adding value to health services and improving a population's health status. Those implications include greater speed in accessing and providing information to consumers and to providers, as well as the use of digital technology to more accurately measure vital signs — and everything else about the human body, feet and all.

18

•

The Evidence Revolution

The meteoric shower of medicine's scientific achievements can overwhelm a doctor's mind. A patient has no assurance that his or her doctor is able to take into account all relevant scientific knowledge and integrate it with the patient's own condition.
— LAWRENCE L. WEED, *BRITISH MEDICAL JOURNAL* (JULY 26, 1997)

The third International Conference on the Scientific Basis of Health Services was held in Toronto, Canada, from October 1 to 3, 1999. Like its two predecessors — the first conference, held in London, England, in 1995, marked a watershed in the evidence-based revolution; the second was held in Amsterdam, the Netherlands, in 1997 — the conference brought together an international, transdisciplinary audience with an interest in integrating and synthesizing evidence and information into major issues in health-care practice, public policy, and health management. Conference sessions explored and challenged the applicability of theory and practice developed outside the health-care arena. The format of the meeting combined plenary and small-group working sessions, interspersed with opportunities for social interaction and networking. An audience of some 600 delegates, representing an international mix of practitioners, clinicians, policy makers, researchers, and managers, attended the conference.

In the past decade, throughout the industrialized world, the evidence revolution has gained momentum in health services. Evidence-based practice is one of the most powerful of the new ideas in health care discussed in Chapter 1. For most of its history, the practice of medicine and the delivery of health-care services have been a matter of clinical observation, trial, and error. It is only with the advent of modern computing that massive randomized clinical trials could be undertaken, and it is only with the processing capacity of modern computers that vast quantities of data could be analyzed for patterns. In the cold scientific light of these studies, much conventional medical wisdom has been found wanting. Many techniques and interventions have been found to be either less effective than previously believed or wholly ineffective.

The evidence revolution pits modern computing and the social sciences against a conventional wisdom. It is a messy contest since, although medicine has conducted itself as a science in the lab, it has conducted itself as a guild in its actual practice (see Chapter 6 for more on the culture of doctors). The evidence-based revolution fundamentally challenges this approach, calling on the medical profession to come out of the Middle Ages and into the twenty-first century. To make the spectacle of this transformation livelier still, many of the high priests of the new temple of evidence-based medicine are themselves doctors.

A Swift and Bloodless Revolution

What form is the evidence revolution taking? There is hardly blood in the streets. Most of the revolutionaries are perched in medical institutes, centres for health policy, and universities, in organizations with such non-revolutionary titles as the Institute for Clinical Evaluative Studies or the Utilization Management Commission. The new science brings together the old field of epidemiology (the study of patterns of disease) and the practical matter of delivering health care, creating a kind of hypercharged clinical epidemiology. Its practitioners apply powerful analytic tools and good statistical science to the delivery of care.

Since the 1960s, the field of evidence-based medicine has burgeoned, making it possible now to deal with some of the complexities of measuring how well particular health-care practices actually work.

"The speed of the increase in our knowledge about efficacy is astonishing," pronounced Dr. Mark Chassin, chair of the Department of Health Policy of the Mount Sinai School of Medicine in New York City, in an interview. "To be sure, a great deal of what we do in health care cannot be related to a strong scientific foundation, but the fraction that can be has increased dramatically. This will have profound effects on every aspect of health care, from education of future physicians to current physicians' practices, as well as for the organization, financing, and delivery of care," continued Dr. Chassin. "For example, the apprenticeship mode of medical training is giving way to the teaching of lifetime learning skills. The old rules aren't possible anymore."

As I mentioned when introducing this idea in Chapter 1, the silicon chip has enabled the analysis of huge quantities of health data. The results of these analyses are the "evidence" of the evidence-based revolution — and the source of much new thinking. The notion of evidence-based health services has a strong appeal for those paying the bills and those managing budgets. In a world of limited funding for health services, evidence-based practice offers a way of deciding where to direct funds so they do the most good based on science, not politics, tradition, or trial and error. Some advocates of evidence-based policy may believe it can be a substitute for rationing, while others view it as a means of rationing. In my view, better evidence as a basis for decision making will simply improve outcomes, full stop.

The "holy grail" of evidence-based advocates is influence on clinical practice. Merely undertaking research is not enough; it has value only insofar as it actually changes how health-care services are managed and delivered, in the view of the evidence-based community. Without strong links between research and practice, two solitudes exist; research remains within the academic domain, while managers and policy makers remain focused on solving the latest public crises.

Quality

Managed care, with its principal emphasis on obtaining price discounts from physicians and hospitals, has not addressed the issue of quality, according to Dr. Chassin. But if this issue is not addressed, the pressure on costs can only increase; the way to reduce these pressures over the long term is to focus on *proven* quality in health care.

In Dr. Chassin's view, three kinds of quality problems exist in our health-care systems: underuse, overuse, and misuse. "If we fix overuse or misuse problems, we improve quality and reduce costs at the same time. Overuse is ubiquitous in American medicine, from the simplest things we do to the most complicated surgical interventions. Speaking conservatively, we could safely eliminate 20% of what we do in health care, and quality would improve."

However, he cautions, "if we want to get a handle on inappropriate use, we are going to have to rely on more than the scientific evidence in the literature. The problem is the will to examine this issue." If inappropriate use accounts for even only 20% of health-care money spent, the stakes are enormous. In a hospital the size of Mount Sinai, about 2,000 patients are injured every year through the inappropriate use of drugs; about one-third of these injuries are preventable — and they are expensive. "Each one of these adverse drug events adds about $2,000 (U.S.) to an admission."

As in so many other areas, "we are starting to learn that if you do it the right way the first time, it also turns out to be the least expensive way of reducing costs — rather than screwing things up and fixing it. We are just at the leading edge of improving outcomes and efficiencies."

Dr. Chassin added that, if overuse and misuse were eliminated, costs could be controlled without the need for rationing.

One of the key challenges for the evidence-based movement at the clinical level is connecting with the movement to better inform and empower citizens as consumers. The consumer movement shares the objective of better outcomes. But the evidence-based movement has been focused largely on health providers, and, to a lesser degree, it has sought to influence policy makers. However, it would seem to have a natural ally in the new health consumerism, with its focus on better information for patients leading to more effective behaviour. What is evidence, after all, but better information transformed into evidence through research?

The British concept of the Patient Charter is at the leading edge of this field. The idea of a "consumer-transparent" set of benchmarks is a radical change in health care. Introduced in 1992, these charters apply to both public- and private-sector health care. Later, after hospital standards — the league tables described in Chapter 15 — were implemented, the Patient Charters were extended to include primary care. They cover fifty-nine measures, including waiting times for:

◇ emergency-room care
◇ hip surgery
◇ cardiac surgery

Cochrane Collaboration

Archie Cochrane led an eventful life. From his student days at Cambridge to his role in the Spanish Civil War as a member of the International Brigade, then later as prisoner of war, and still later as a medical officer in Crete, Archie Cochrane followed his beliefs.

One of the leading intellectual lights of the outcomes movement, Professor Cochrane, for whom the British Cochrane Centres are named, was a British medical researcher who contributed greatly to the development of the science of epidemiology. His 1972 book, *Effectiveness and*

Efficiency: Random Reflections on Health Services, inspired health researchers to apply scientific evidence gained from randomized clinical trials to decision making. He wrote in 1979, "It is surely a great criticism of our profession that we have not organized a critical summary by speciality or sub-speciality, adapted periodically, of all relevant randomized controlled trials."

The Cochrane Collaboration, named for this tireless patient advocate, an international group of 77 health researchers from 11 countries, was formed in response to Dr. Cochrane's call for systematic, up-to-date reviews of relevant randomized clinical trials of health care. (Randomized clinical trials are acknowledged as the best method of determining the outcome of medical interventions. They compare the outcome of a treatment with the experience of a similar group of patients not treated.)

Cochrane's suggestion that the methods used to prepare and maintain reviews of controlled trials in pregnancy and childbirth should be applied more widely was taken up by the research program of the National Health Service in the United Kingdom. Funds were provided to establish a Cochrane Centre, which would collaborate with other similar centres in the United Kingdom and elsewhere, to facilitate systematic reviews of randomized controlled trials across all areas of health care.

When the first Cochrane Centre was opened in Oxford, in October 1992, those involved expressed the hope that there would be a collaborative international response to Cochrane's agenda. This idea was outlined at a meeting organized six months later by the New York Academy of Sciences. In October 1993 — at what was to become the first in a series of annual Cochrane Colloquia — seventy-seven medical experts from nine countries co-founded the "Cochrane Collaboration."

The Cochrane Collaboration has evolved rapidly since then, but its basic objectives and principles have remained the same. It aims to help people make well-informed decisions about health care by preparing, maintaining, and ensuring the accessibility of systematic reviews of the effects of various medical interventions. The collaboration is built on eight principles:

◇ collaboration;

◇ building on the enthusiasm of individuals;

◇ avoiding duplication;

◇ minimizing bias;

◇ keeping up to date;

◇ ensuring relevance;

◇ ensuring access; and

◇ continually improving the quality of its work.

Cochrane Reviews (the principal output of the collaboration) are published electronically in successive issues of *The Cochrane Database of Systematic Reviews*. Preparation and maintenance of Cochrane Reviews are the responsibility of international collaborative review groups. At the beginning of 1997, more than forty existing and planned review groups covered most of the important areas of health care. For example:

◇ How can stroke and its effects be prevented and treated?

◇ What drugs should be used to prevent and treat malaria, tuberculosis, and other important infectious diseases?

◇ What strategies are effective in preventing brain and spinal-cord injury and its consequences, and what rehabilitative measures can help those with residual disabilities?

Each group is responsible for reviewing, in a scientific and systematic way, information on the efficacy of treatment in its particular area. This information is carefully analyzed. The group then writes a formal, structured report, which is published electronically. (See the following chart.) The process is repeated as necessary to keep the reviews current.

The members of these groups — researchers, health-care professionals, consumers, and others — share an interest in generating reliable, up-to-date evidence relevant to the prevention, treatment, and rehabilitation of particular health problems or groups of problems.

Each collaborative review group prepares a plan outlining how it will

The Systematic Review Process: Cochrane Style

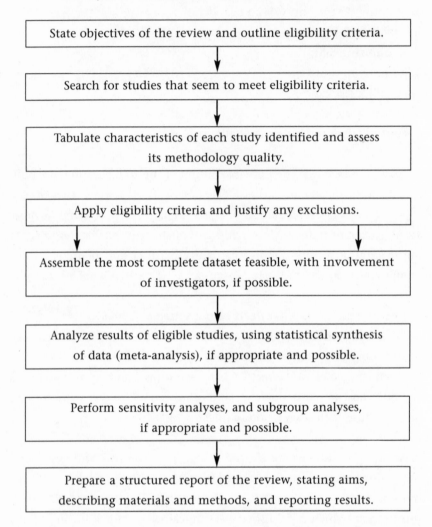

State objectives of the review and outline eligibility criteria.

Search for studies that seem to meet eligibility criteria.

Tabulate characteristics of each study identified and assess its methodology quality.

Apply eligibility criteria and justify any exclusions.

Assemble the most complete dataset feasible, with involvement of investigators, if possible.

Analyze results of eligible studies, using statistical synthesis of data (meta-analysis), if appropriate and possible.

Perform sensitivity analyses, and subgroup analyses, if appropriate and possible.

Prepare a structured report of the review, stating aims, describing materials and methods, and reporting results.

contribute to the Collaboration's objectives. This plan, developed in consultation with the staff of one or more Cochrane Centres (which collectively share responsibility for coordinating the development of the Collaboration), must be based on agreements reached at exploratory meetings of those interested in becoming involved in the group. The plan defines the scope that the group will take on and the specific topics falling within this scope. It describes who will have responsibility for planning, coordinating, and monitoring the group's work (a coordinating editor, supported by an editorial team). The group identifies and assembles in a specialized register as high a proportion as possible of all the studies relevant to its declared scope; various members, drawing on the studies in the register, take responsibility for preparing and maintaining various reviews. Every group appoints an individual, based in the same place as the coordinating editor, to organize and manage the day-to-day activities of the group.

Members of collaborative review groups receive support in tackling these various tasks through training materials developed by the Collaboration, and through training workshops organized by Cochrane Centres (and sometimes by the groups themselves). Whenever possible, training for people preparing and maintaining Cochrane Reviews is, not surprisingly, based on the results of empirical research.

The Cochrane Collaboration Web site can be found at www.som.finc. flinders.edu.ca/FUSA/Cochrane

The Evidence Revolution Around the World

In the United Kingdom, the chief revolutionary of the evidence- or outcomes-based movement has been Professor Michael Peckham. As director of research for the National Health Service in the mid-1990s, Peckham convinced its executive that they needed to spend 1.5% of their total budget, or £240 million per year, on research. Not basic scientific research, not looking for a new cure or technique, but rather research on how to better manage the health system — on what is working and what is not.

The fact that the first international conference on evidence-based medicine was held in London, England, represented something of the triumph of Professor Peckham's tremendous efforts to promote this cause.

In Canada, Dr. Henry Friesen, head of the Medical Research Council, has presided over a major change of course as that research-funding body now seeks to place greater emphasis on applied research in the health services.

The health-services revolution has taken hold in a host of countries, from Australia to South Africa.

Denial and Resistance

As research centres spring up, funded by governments or health maintenance organizations, they run into resistance from the mainstream of the medical profession. Their work is seen as not only a challenge to conventional wisdom but also as an implicit criticism of how physicians practise medicine. Many working physicians advance a number of arguments against this outcomes revolution.

First and foremost, they argue that it is different to statistically measure a series of cases than to be there at the point of care. Faced with a child in pain and the danger of a rupturing appendix, a physician is inclined to, and in fact is obligated to, do everything he or she can to help; if a certain treatment seems most likely to be the child's best bet, how can anyone in good conscience assign her to the "control" group that does not get it? Another oft-heard argument is that the statistical bases used by outcomes-based advocates simply are not capturing enough data to be useful.

Although there is some validity to each of these arguments, the overwhelming weight of evidence suggests that we can, in fact, learn from this kind of research — that as medicine seeks to become a full science, it needs to embrace, not reject, what clinical epidemiologists have to contribute. Enlightened leaders in the medical profession are increasingly advocates of outcomes-based analyses, so long as they are conducted in a thorough, scientific manner.

As more and more clinical protocols driven by evidence are implemented, we are also seeing a subtle use of evidence at the point of care. With enough data, choices can be made in a more sophisticated way. For example, for a number of years a debate raged over two drugs used to treat heart attack. Massive randomized studies were financed by pharmaceutical companies eager to break in with their new and more expensive products. Streptokinase, the old treatment, came into direct competition with TPA (tissue plasminogen activator), the new, bioengineered treatment. At first the issue turned on which drug was "better." Hospitals, pushed by medical staff to use the more expensive TPA, rebelled when the first evidence came in showing that it had no greater effectiveness. Later evidence has shown greater effectiveness — in certain populations. The end result in leading centres has been a more careful use of *both* medications — that is, the use of a protocol that indicates to the physician when TPA has advantages and when streptokinase would be equally effective.

In the expanding world of pharmaco-economics, it will be essential to know not only whether a drug is good or bad, but in precisely which cases it is the appropriate drug, and what the alternatives are for the other cases.

Thus, cost-effectiveness comes into the equation as well. Fundamentally, consumers and payers are asking, "If this is the most cost-effective solution, will it work? Is there a less expensive way of getting an equally good result?" Economics has come to health care, aided and abetted by the outcomes movement; it will not be leaving at any predictable point in the future.

Health Indicators

Two years ago I agreed to become the volunteer board chair of the Canadian Institute for Health Information. One of our main priorities is to develop a set of indicators to measure and track the health of Canadians. Dr. John Miller, a respected leader in public health, has been spearheading the institute's efforts to determine what measurements to use.

A consensus conference in the spring of 1999 led to a broad plan of indicators. The categories have not all been matched with specific measurements, but the outline of a set of indicators is becoming clear. It is grouped into four clusters, as shown in the tables on pages 253–55: health status, non-medical determinants of health, health-system performance, and community and health-system characteristics.

In addition to these four clusters of indicators, some others were also identified by the participants in the conference for future development; see the table on pages 256–57. Over time, through consultation, more indicators will be added under each of the headings.

Conclusions

Evidence has a new ally: digital technologies, with their remarkable ability to scan vast mountains of data, searching for patterns. Efforts to study the studies, such as the Cochrane Collaboration, offer a firm foundation for improved clinical practice. But is it being oversold? Are we committing the same error that we did in our endless quest for the magic bullet, the miracle cure for cancer, seeking a new panacea in the outcomes movement?

Evidence is not a panacea. All of the shortcomings of health systems will not be solved by better evidence. Still, it will help. It is the interaction of better evidence and a more open, informed process between doctors, nurses, and patients that will lead to true improvements.

Evidence is a powerful tool. Placed in the hands of the existing guilds of medicine and nursing, it will improve clinical practice. Placed in the hands of the public — patients, taxpayers, and citizens — it will lead to profound changes in the speed and quality of health services. A more informed public is an inevitable consequence of television, the digital age, and higher levels of education.

The tension between evidence and historical practice will result in transformations, both big and little, in relationships. Patients will become, in more ways, consumers. Physicians will become advisers to patients, aiding them in navigating the tricky shoals of expanding treatment options. Nurses will also take on new roles in patient education.

I was an early, strong devotee of the evidence-based movement, and I remain convinced of its overall merit. The difficult challenge is to gain the confidence of providers, be they physicians, nurses, pharmacists, or others. With their involvement, evidence can lead to new and better care for patients.

Health Indicators Confirmed at the 1999 CIHI Consensus Conference

Health Status

Deaths	Health Conditions	Human Function	Well-Being
• infant mortality	• overweight*	• functional health	• self-rated health
• perinatal deaths	• arthritis	• disability days*	• self-rated "excellent health for two consecutive years"
• life expectancy	• diabetes	• activity limitation	• self-esteem
• circulatory deaths	• asthma	• health expectancy	• mastery
• cancer deaths	• chronic pain*		
• respiratory deaths	• depression*		
• suicide	• injury hospitalizations		
• unintentional-injury deaths	• food/water-borne diseases		
• pertussis deaths*			
• AIDS deaths*			
• potential years of life lost (<75)			
• inequality in life expectancy*			

Source for tables on pages 253–57: Canadian Institute for Health Information Conference proceedings, 1999.

Health Indicators Confirmed at the 1999 CIHI Consensus Conference (cont'd)

Non-Medical Determinants of Health

Health Behaviours	Living and Working Conditions	Personal Resources	Environmental Factors
• smoking rate	• high school and post-secondary graduation	• school readiness	• yet to be confirmed
• youth smoking rate	• unemployment rate	• social support	
• smoking initiation (average age*)	• long-term and youth unemployment	• life stress	
• regular heavy drinking	• low-income rate		
• physical activity	• children in low-income families		
• breast-feeding	• income inequality		
	• housing affordability		
	• crime rate and youth crime rate		
	• decision latitude at work*		

Community and Health-System Characteristics

• population count	• doctors and nurses per capita	• heart bypass rates
• teen pregnancy*/ teen births*	• hospital stays per capita (possibly by duration of stay)*	• hip replacement
• expenditures per capita		• knee replacement
		• hysterectomy

Health-System Performance

Acceptability	Accessibility	Appropriateness	Competence
• yet to be determined	• influenza immunization, 65+	• vaginal birth after Caesarean section	
	• screening mammography, age 50–69	• breast-conserving surgery	
	• Pap smears, age 18–69	• Caesarean sections	
	• childhood immunizations**		• hip fractures
	• quitting smoking	• surgical day-case rates	
	• low birth weight	• may not require hospitalization	
	• pertussis, measles, tuberculosis	• % non-hospital days	
	• HIV	• expected compared to actual stay	
	• chlamydia		
	• pneumonia and influenza hospitalizations		
	• deaths due to medically treatable diseases		

* Based on feedback from the conference, proposed indicators are under review for feasibility, comparability, availability of data; some indicators are also under review for significant proposed changes in definition.

** Limited data available.

Other Health Indicators for Future Development

Health Status			
Deaths	**Health Conditions**	**Human Function**	**Well-Being**
• smoking-attributable deaths	• work injuries	• functional health	• sense of coherence
	• prevalance of dementia	• disability days	
	• hepatitis C	• health expectancy	
	• cancer incidence		

Non-Medical Determinants of Health			
Health Behaviours	**Living and Working Conditions**	**Personal Resources**	**Environmental Factors**
• dietary practices	• percent of children "in care"	• literacy rates	• exposure to second-hand smoke
• bicycle-helmet use	• homelessness	• caregiver burden	• air quality
• condom use	• number of "working poor"		• water quality
• protection from sun	• housing quality		• toxic waste
• seat-belt use	• community cohesion		• ecological footprint
• driving after drinking			

Other Health Indicators for Future Development (cont'd)

Community and Health-System Characteristics	
• cultural diversity	• cost per weighted case
• availability of licensed child-care spaces	• magnetic resonance imaging (MRI)
• labour-force participation rates	

19

•

Disease-State Management

Early experience suggests that disease management can lead to demonstrably better outcomes, as measured by clinical results, cost, and patient satisfaction.

— BOSTON CONSULTING GROUP (1995)

One of the most intriguing directions of health care at the dawn of the millennium is the concept of disease-state management. This idea, which is largely being pursued in the United States, is based on the hypothesis that, rather than managing *episodes* of illness, it would be more effective to organize a system of intervention to manage the *whole course* of a disease. Variations on this approach, often under other names, are under way in many parts of the U.S. health system. Many jurisdictions, however, lack the robust information technology needed to support a full program of disease-state management.

The Boston Consulting Group provided a working definition in a 1995 paper called "The Promise of Disease Management." Their view was that patient care would be redefined by this new organizing concept:

> Disease management is an approach to patient care that coordinates resources across the entire health-care delivery system and throughout the life cycle of a disease. Traditional approaches focus mainly on discrete medical episodes, attempting to minimize the expense of individual cost components, including physician services, pharmaceuticals, and hospitalization. Disease management takes a more systemic approach, focusing on the patient with a disease as the relevant unit of management, with an emphasis on quality as well as cost.
>
> The three primary elements of disease management are:
>
> — A knowledge base that quantifies the economic structure of the disease and describes care guidelines (what care should be provided, by whom, and in what setting) for discrete patient segments;
> — A delivery system of health-care professionals and organizations, closely coordinating to provide care throughout the course of a disease, breaking down traditional boundaries between medical specialties and institutions; and
> — A continuous improvement process that measures clinical behaviour, refines treatment standards, and improves the quality of care provided.

How does disease-state management work? Consider the treatment of diabetes, for example. When you think of diabetes treatment, you probably think immediately of the drug insulin. In the United States, some $500 million (U.S.) a year is spent on insulin, which allows diabetics to function and live; however, the total direct medical costs of treating diabetes in the United States is estimated to be $44 billion a year, or nearly

90 times the amount spent on insulin. In other words, insulin constitutes only 1% of the total cost of treating diabetes, when hospital days
and all other costs are considered. Fifteen million Americans live with
diabetes — and even today, many die from it. Some statistics on this disease are shown in the table below.

Total Health-Care Burden of Diabetes, United States

Total Patients (U.S.)	15.7 million
Type I	800,000
Type II	9.5 million diagnosed; 5.4 million undiagnosed
New Cases (annually)	13,000, Type I; 800,000, Type II
Related Deaths (annually)	193,000 (sixth leading cause of death in the United States)
Cost	$44 billion (U.S.) annually in direct medical costs $54 billion more for premature death and disability
Treatments	Type I: careful diet control and insulin injections; Type II: diet, exercise, drugs — such as Glucophage and Rezulin — and insulin

Source: Alexandra Alger, "Decoding Diabetes," *Forbes*, June 14, 1999.

A disease-state management approach to diabetes would focus on *all* of
the interventions and activities available for treating this disease, linking
together in one package not only the drug and its delivery vehicle, but
diet and counselling, hospitalizations, disability, etc., and to try to manage all aspects of the illness according to the best available thinking in
an organized way. For example, we know that with diabetes, as with
many other illnesses, compliance with the treatment regimen is a major
factor affecting treatment outcome. So more resources might be directed
toward finding ways compliance can be improved — such as better infor-

mation, telephone follow-up, and self-monitoring.

Some $300 million (U.S.) per year of venture-capital money was poured into various approaches to U.S. disease-state management in the early and mid-1990s. This potential opportunity captured the imagination of drug makers, who felt caught between more demanding markets and the growing size of the investment needed to bring a new drug to market (see Chapter 8). The drug makers reasoned that they could, instead of devoting all of their efforts to invent, say, a new form of insulin, work out how to save consumers' health and payers' money by better managing the $50-billion cost of the disease, in addition to fighting for a share of the $500-million-per-annum diabetes health-services market. Disease-state management is not necessarily an altruistic aim; there are profits to be earned for pharmaceutical companies. A disease-state management program represents a way of selling intellectual property about a disease, separate from the drug developed to treat it.

It is not just drug makers but also leading health-care providers, such as the Mayo Clinic and others, that are interested in taking their particular expertise and packaging it in different ways for different markets. So, too, firms with a special interest in various diseases are moving forward. Will disease-state management be another health-care fad to fail and be forgotten? Or will it become the dominant approach to care in the twenty-first century? Only time will tell, but my belief is that the techniques of disease-state management represent an important, permanent advance.

The Scope of Disease-State Management

Disease-state management is applicable to a range of medical problems, but it will likely play an especially important role in coping with chronic illness. As populations age in the industrialized world, many acute illnesses are now being managed through a combination of therapies as long-term, chronic conditions. In these areas, disease-state management has a chance of making a radical difference in both the quality and cost of care.

The following charts show the disease groups viewed as most able to benefit from a disease-state management approach:

Candidates for Disease-State Management

Asthma

Problem

- Some patients are undiagnosed and undermedicated, leading to high rates of ER admission and hospitalization.

Disease-Management Approach

- evaluation of patients for asthma; classification as mild, moderate, and severe
- management of critical junctures for each asthma segment
- use of database to monitor outcomes and refine process

Results

- primary-care visits up 200%
- drug use up 100% for mild asthmatics, down 33% in moderate/severe segments
- hospital days down 25%, ER admissions reduced by 20%
- total cost for asthma population down 30% from trend line

Diabetes

Problem

- Patients do not optimally monitor and manage blood-sugar levels, leading to serious, but avoidable, complications.

Disease-Management Approach

- interdisciplinary teams of primary-care physicians and specialists, supported by nutritionists and podiatrists
- self-monitoring of blood glucose
- education programs
- automation of medical records with clinically driven "ticklers" (reminders) to ensure appropriate care

Results

- fewer hospital admissions
- fewer medical complications
- higher quality of life

Candidates for Disease-State Management (cont'd)

Congestive Heart Failure (CHF)

Problem

- High-risk patients are not managed adequately in the outpatient setting, leading to premature deterioration that requires hospitalization.

Disease-Management Approach

- CHF clinics staffed by specially trained cardiologists
- specialized cardiac home-care nurses to identify early signs of deconditioning
- algorithm-based telemanagement
- cardiac rehabilitation

Results

- 50% to 60% decrease in hospital admissions
- 40% to 45% improvement in functional status
- decreased mortality

HIV Disease

Problem

- Many patients receive poor care from MDs unfamiliar with HIV and use hospital resources unnecessarily.

Disease-Management Approach

- direction of patients to HIV specialists
- specialized HIV RNs to answer patient calls and provide home visits on a twenty-four-hour basis
- pharmaceutical compliance management

Results

- home-care costs increase up to 6 times
- reduce hospitalization by up to 75%
- reduce total cost by up to 50%

Source: *New England Journal of Medicine*, 33 1995: 1190–95.

The disease-state management approach will manifest itself most rapidly in the United States. There, health systems and HMOs will be approached by disease-state managers offering so-called disease carve-outs — that is, for a fixed sum of money per patient, the disease-state manager will look after a defined population. This will be an appealing pitch, providing the service can be delivered competently, because it will give health systems a predictable set of outcomes, as well as predictable costs, for potentially expensive populations.

Much of our ability to manage disease states is again driven by computer technology, particularly the information storage and manipulation that could be achieved by much faster chips.

Tools and Support Structures

Combining key tools with the appropriate infrastructure results in an effective process for managing a population's health. The goal is an organized set of programs capable of improving people's health before they are acutely ill. The focus is on early diagnosis of risk with links to wellness programs. For those with chronic diseases, the real power of an effective program is case management with strategic interventions, which can be as simple as a phone call to remind a patient to take a medication. Taken together, these initiatives can improve the health of a population by improving the health of those most at risk of illness.

Tools and Support Structures for Disease-State Management

Tools	Support Structures
• patient segmentation, screening, and tracking	• information technology
• preventive/wellness programs	• case management
• patient education	• home-based services
• comprehensive clinical guidelines	• data-collection systems/services
• patient quality-of-life satisfaction monitoring	• telemedicine/telephone/ RN triage
• outcomes measurement/reporting	

Source: APM, Inc. Presentation 14804a78, October 13, 1996.

Population Health

Another way of looking at disease-state management is by placing it in the spectrum of health approaches. Disease-state management focuses on groups of patients with the same disease. This places it somewhere between narrower case-by-case efforts and broader health programs directed at the entire population.

From Individuals to Populations

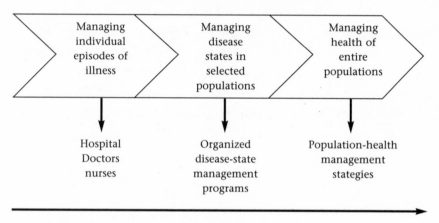

Source: APM, Inc. Presentation 14804a78, October 13, 1996.

Conclusions

As with many innovations in health care, the early promise of disease-state management appears to have been oversold. An excellent concept and worthy approach met three formidable obstacles: first, the concept works best with a handful of major chronic diseases, such as asthma and diabetes. Trying to apply it to every medical circumstance is folly. Second, to make the concept work, robust information technology to track both patients and interventions is essential. Without strong data and highly organized intervention programs, either telephone- or clinic-based, disease management enjoys only modest results. Finally, disease-state management emerged as a concept in the contentious world of managed care. Many groups concerned with specific diseases, groups that should have been allies in the search for a better process of care, have not been enthusiastic. Why? Disease-state management, with its seeking of optimal care, was viewed by many as a means of reducing care, and was therefore resisted. The use of disease-state management by pharma companies as a marketing tool did not help its reputation.

Time, greater sophistication in health-information systems, and a better communication of the benefits of this approach will allow disease-state management an important role in the future health system. Giving a much more powerful role to patients in the disease-state management process is a solid route to achieving its full potential; if they are linked to self-care, the techniques of disease-state management offer a potent means of improving care, health status, and outcomes.

20

•

Human Genetics: The Final Frontier

This is more important than putting a man on the moon or split-ting the atom. Biomedical research will be divided into what we did before we had the human genome and what we did after.

— DR. FRANCIS COLLINS, DIRECTOR, HUMAN GENOME PROJECT, NATIONAL INSTITUTES OF HEALTH

The Human Genome Project is one of the most ambitious research undertakings in scientific history. It seems that newspaper headlines trumpet the discovery of new genes every week, some of them linked to human disease. As rapidly as the genes are discovered, diagnostic-testing techniques based on this new research are being developed. Gene therapies to ultimately treat these diseases are also evolving, making this decade one of the most exciting in the history of genetic research.

All these complex therapies are dependent on our growing ability to understand and alter DNA. For those whose high-school biology is distant — or never existed in the first place — I offer below a short primer in genetics and DNA as a background to how this fascinating topic fits into the world of health care.

Genetics 101

Our genes — we each have more than 50,000 of them — are contained in the chromosomes stored in each of our cells. You can think of a gene as a specific section of a chromosome, or as a stretch of DNA. The fundamental set of genes that defines an organism is called the genome. Your DNA stores the blueprint, or instruction set, for creating you.

DNA is like genetic software. But unlike most software products, which are constantly being upgraded, DNA is permanent. You cannot change the DNA with which you were born; it remains immutable as you grow from the single cell that began your existence into a complex organism with specialized cells that go on to fight infections, repair wounds, and create the children of the next generation.

We are limited by our DNA. That is why cats never give birth to puppies, and oak trees never sprout from pine cones. The ancient genetic observation is that "like makes like." Yet two of the same sort of pine tree growing in different environments, or twins raised in two different circumstances may turn out to be very different from one another. The genome determines the basics, but how an organism develops is influenced by circumstances.

Genes and Disease

Some diseases are genetic disorders. Certain genes, if inherited, inevitably lead to a disorder such as hemophilia, cystic fibrosis, Huntington's chorea, or muscular dystrophy. These are usually the result of mutations in one gene. Hundreds of human genetic diseases are attributable to single-gene defects (some of the more common ones are listed below). We actually know quite a bit about these types of inherited diseases, which are relatively easy research targets.

In other cases, inheriting certain genes leads to a predisposition, or an increased susceptibility, to a disease. Hypertension, atherosclerosis, heart disease, most cancers, and some mental illnesses fall into this category. Predispositions, which often result from the interplay among several genes, are much more complicated to study. Different families may have quite different mutations, for one thing. For another, environmental factors, such as diet, smoking, drinking, or viral infections, also influence the onset of these diseases. The more that scientists learn about our genes, the more quickly they can map new ones.

Accurate diagnosis is essential to medical progress. Biochemical and molecular clues are increasingly important in helping doctors identify and treat diseases ever more precisely. Once a gene is located and its DNA sequence determined, scientists can develop a test for the presence of the gene in a patient. There may be several forms of some diseases, each caused by a different defective gene. A drug that works well on a patient with one defective gene may not work on a patient with a different one.

With appropriate screening and counselling, people in families that have a history of certain disorders can determine whether or not they carry the defective genes. This allows them to make intelligent reproductive decisions based on more complete information. People who know they have a genetic predisposition to certain genetic conditions can receive counselling, and take steps to delay or prevent the disease.

Family studies showed scientists that certain genes are "linked," i.e., inherited together. But it is only recently that scientific advances have allowed us to discover their actual physical location, or chromosome position. Historically, the first genes to be physically mapped were on the X chromosome, one of the two that determines a person's sex. Eventually, methods were developed that allowed scientists to assign genes to any one specific chromosome, and finally to specific sites on the chromosomes, making the Human Genome Project possible.

Applications for Gene-Related Research

Heart disease, a leading killer in industrialized countries, has many different causes. Inherited traits interact with environmental influences such as diet, fat, exercise, smoking, and other, still-unknown factors. Treating heart disease properly depends on an understanding of these causes.

Among the inherited traits that affect a person's chances of contracting heart disease is the way the body handles, or metabolizes, fats. A variety of genes are involved in making, using, transporting, and disposing of fats and cholesterol. Some genes make proteins that carry fats around the body; others make enzymes that break fats down or convert them into other substances. All it takes is one or two metabolic roadblocks, and a person can end up with blood vessels that are easily clogged with fats — an outcome that can often be avoided with adjustments to diet.

Inherited traits that contribute to heart-disease risk can be identified in approximately 80% of heart-disease patients. An increasingly clear picture of the genes and processes involved is emerging. People with specific traits respond differently to various treatments. Diet, drug, and exercise therapy must be individualized in order to achieve the best outcome for any patient; there's no one-size-fits-all treatment. About half of the close relatives of heart patients have the same genetic trait. Risk identification can prevent or delay the onset of disease, or lessen its effects.

Mental and nervous system disorders also have a genetic basis. There has long been recognition that alcoholism, certain mental disorders, and other conditions involving the nervous system tend to occur more often in some families than in others. Identification of the genes responsible for many of these problems is under way.

Receptors, and their variations, also play a role in determining responsiveness to some antipsychotic medications and drugs used in treating Parkinson disease. As with any other type of disorder, knowing which genes are causing or influencing the condition can lead to better diagnosis and treatment.

This ability to home in on a more precise diagnosis, leading to better decisions regarding treatment, is the major benefit of genetic research for health care.

Cancer: A More Complex Case

Cancer is the major cause of death in the world's developed countries; one in five cancer patients dies within five years of first diagnosis. Amazingly, cancer treatments have not changed substantially since the early 1950s. Because it is not a single disease but a complex combination of several different cellular processes gone awry, the way cancer manifests itself varies considerably from person to person.

Benign and malignant tumours also differ at the microscopic level. Benign tumours retain many of the cellular features of the tissue from which they arise. Malignant tumours tend to display a wide range of cell shapes, sizes, and cellular features that do not necessarily reflect their tissue of origin.

Cancer is a genetic disease. Researchers have known for decades that certain cancers seemed to be more prevalent in some families and in some ethnic groups. But even with this strong evidence of a genetic predisposition, cancer was not formally recognized as a genetic disease until the 1980s, when a susceptibility gene for small-cell cancer of the lung was mapped to chromosome three. Now it is generally accepted that cancer arises from the accumulation of mutations in a number of genes responsible for controlling normal cell growth and development. The fact that most environmental carcinogens are mutagens supports the idea of a genetic basis for cancer.

These mutations may be inherited or acquired. They may increase the chances of cancer arising, or initiate it directly. While the chaos that is cancer is always the result of genetic foul-ups, a combination of environmental, dietary, and lifestyle-related factors serve as triggers.

Key Diseases with Genetic Links

Genetic research won't solve all our health problems, but the number of areas where it is promising is large. The following list shows just a few of the diseases that are linked to single-gene disorders:

◇ cystic fibrosis;
◇ fragile X syndrome (a common form of mental retardation);
◇ Huntington chorea;
◇ muscular dystrophy;
◇ sickle-cell anemia; and
◇ Tay-Sachs disease (which causes death through loss of brain cells).

Genetics also offers the hope of breakthroughs in the following diseases, all of which have both genetic and environmental factors (such as diet, smoking, and viruses):

◇ Alzheimer disease;
◇ breast cancer;
◇ colorectal cancer;
◇ coronary-artery disease;
◇ diabetes;
◇ hypertension;
◇ lung cancer;
◇ ovarian cancer;
◇ pancreatic cancer;
◇ Parkinson syndrome; and
◇ prostate cancer.

Genetics and Health Care

Advances in genetic research are applicable to an increasing number of areas of health care. Patients, as well as physicians, are adjusting to the promise of this "new medicine." Once the genes responsible for a disease are pinpointed, scientists can begin to track down the errors that lead to the medical problem. This kind of research is expected to result in new treatments and cures for many diseases, making genetics the star attraction of health-care research that will eventually transform health-care services in many ways.

Delineating the full sequence of human genes is expected to take until 2003. Analyzing this information will continue well into the twenty-first century, and provide a new foundation for biomedical research.

An additional goal of the Human Genome Project is to improve the tools and technologies for exploring DNA.

The effort is already paying off, with gene discoveries at an all-time high. DNA diagnostics are already providing precise diagnoses for an increasing number of conditions. In many cases, the earlier a condition is diagnosed, the better the chances of treating it. Improved treatments are expected to follow for many of these conditions. The information gathered has also been useful for comprehending gene action and evolutionary relationships.

Tissue-specific gene discovery can be a faster route to some discoveries. The goal of the Human Genome Project is completeness — the entire sequence of human DNA. But much of our DNA doesn't code for genes — and of the 50,000 or so genes in any cell, only a fraction — say 3,000 — are expressed, i.e., have a detectable effect on cells. It's that subset of genes that makes a tissue unique and determines whether it's healthy or diseased. So some researchers take a shortcut and look for genes, tissue by tissue. By comparing genes expressed from one tissue to those from another, scientists can tell which genes are unique to a given tissue. Similarly, comparing gene expression between healthy tissues and diseased ones can suggest which genes may be involved in a given disease. Modern biomedical instruments feed sequence information directly into supercomputers (like IBM's Blue Gene — see Chapter 17) capable of processing the information.

Identifying genes can also hasten the discovery of new drugs. The key to developing new medicines lies in the proteins produced by genes. Once researchers identify and isolate a gene likely to be involved in a genetic disease, they can then move the gene into bacteria or yeast cells, which then manufacture the protein at much higher levels than in the original cell. Having the protein in hand can point the way to new pharmaceutical discoveries. Scientists can then study how it interacts and binds with other molecules. Ideally they can discover what role the protein plays in healthy and diseased cells. For instance, if too much of a particular protein causes a disease, then a drug that binds to the protein, inhibiting its impact, might help.

Pandora's Box: What Should
We Do with Genetic Knowledge?

Science is now often in a position to predict how likely a particular couple is to have a child with a certain disorder. This power gives rise to ethical challenges regarding the use of this genetic information. Who should know what, when, and about whom — and who decides this? Who owns commercial rights to use information about genes we all share? Society's understanding of the concepts of health, disease, and normality; of privacy and justice; and of intellectual property and commerce will all play key roles in shaping applications of emerging knowledge about genetics.

Discoverers of potentially informative partial sequences have attempted to claim rights to the future discoveries made by others using those partial sequences. This kind of controversy raises questions about the fairness and efficiency of laws in allocating rewards and incentives along the path of cumulative innovation. Do patents promote commercial investment in product development, or do they interfere with scientific communication and collaboration, retarding the overall research effort? If such information remains in the public domain, accessible to all, will commercial product development be stifled?

Dr. Craig Venter, CEO of Celera Genomics, has promised, "Once we have finished sequencing the entire genetic code we will make it available for free to every scientist on the planet over the Internet." In the search for therapeutics, genetic prospectors are sampling plant and animal species from tropical forests. What are the responsibilities of genetic prospectors to the peoples or countries from which their discoveries come? These are just some of the questions that scientists, corporations, government agencies, and others are debating as we enter the genetic era.

Who Should Be Tested?

When does it help to know if you carry a mutation? The broadest, most basic answer is "when you can do something about it." In many cases, medical researchers have not bridged the gap between their ability to predict and diagnose conditions and their ability to prevent, treat, or cure them.

Genetic testing can take many forms. Some of the most prevalent are as follows:

◇ Carrier Identification — Couples whose families have a history of recessive genetic disorders and who are considering having children may opt for this kind of testing. Three common disorders with carrier-identification tests are cystic fibrosis, Tay-Sachs disease, and sickle-cell anemia.

◇ Prenatal Diagnosis — Genetic testing of a fetus may be desirable when there is a risk of bearing a child with genes associated with mental retardation or certain other disorders. Down syndrome is one of the most common genetic conditions screened for by this method.

◇ Newborn Screening — Frequently conducted as preventive health measures, these tests usually offer clear benefits because treatments exist. Testing for phenylketonuria and congenital hypothyroidism is common.

◇ Late-Onset Disorders — Many adult diseases, such as cancer and heart disease, are complex, and have both genetic and environmental causes. Testing may indicate a susceptibility or predisposition for these problems. Some "simple" diseases caused by single genes, such as Huntington's chorea (for which there is no treatment), are also seen later in life. Testing for these disorders can take place any time; the decision usually hinges on such factors as whether the individual is showing symptoms, whether he or she has any concerns about having children, and whether there is a treatment available.

When to test someone for a genetic disorder is a complex question. It depends on the specifics of the condition in question, on the individual's family and health history, etc. With the exception of some types of newborn screening, widespread genetic screening of everyone for every testable disease would be expensive and time-consuming and would generate little benefit. It would also invade privacy. Usually a set of symptoms, a family history, or some other evidence prompts the question of whether or not to test.

Ultimately, it is the patient who must decide. First, patients must understand the risks, benefits, effectiveness, and alternatives to testing, so they can make an informed decision. Since these tests can be done with a small amount of blood, some people worry that they might be tested without their consent. They need to feel confident that ethical and legal safeguards in the health system will prevent unauthorized testing.

Ensuring the privacy of genetic information is another important concern. Patients, consumer advocates, doctors, legislators, and others are concerned that genetic information could be used to discriminate against carriers of some genetic traits. Losing access to health care is the primary fear in the United States; if your genes suggest a predisposition to certain disorders, will you be considered too expensive to treat? First Lady Hillary Clinton joked at the launch of the Human Genome Project that soon everyone would be uninsurable. Thus, the legislative focus in the early 1990s was almost exclusively on attempting to forbid insurers from using such information in underwriting decisions. Additional concerns include fear of genetic discrimination in employment and in areas such as life insurance.

When the first genetic tests became available, some geneticists predicted a strong patient demand. To date, however, there has been no stampede to get tested. People may not want to know what is in their genes. Some see no point in knowing whether they are carriers of a disease until they contemplate having children. In some cases, lack of education is a barrier: patients — and their physicians — may not understand the testing options. In other cases, the previously mentioned concerns about privacy and genetic discrimination prevent people from getting tested.

From Treatments to Cures: Gene Therapy

Seeking new drugs and treatments is a noble goal, but patients often have to take even the most successful drugs as long as they have the condition it combats — perhaps for an entire lifetime. Finding cures, therefore, is even better. So, instead of trying to counteract bad genes, why not repair or replace them? That's the idea behind gene therapy: DNA becomes a pharmaceutical.

Not all conditions are equally amenable to gene therapy. It's easier to envision replacing a missing gene function than to envision turning off a malfunctioning gene, for example. But even replacing some kinds of absent gene function can be tricky. Inborn metabolic problems, such as a missing enzyme, are the easiest conditions to imagine curing this way.

So far, scientists are only considering somatic-cell gene therapy, which affects only the patient. The ethical considerations of germ-line gene therapy have yet to be fully addressed. "Correcting" a germ-line means making a genetic alteration in an early embryo that affects not only that individual but also all of its descendants. It's been done in lab animals; but applying this level of genetic interference to people is another matter, both scientifically and ethically.

Conclusions

Genetic technology has vast potential socioeconomic repercussions for individuals as well as society. No one wants to spawn a genetic underclass, or a society based on "genetic determinism," in which human beings are judged by their DNA. Genetic testing has the potential to be an invaluable tool, and with appropriate measures to prevent abuse and misuse of genetic information its promise can be fulfilled.

The staggering potential of human genetics is clear. Less transparent is the timeline on which benefits to actual patients are likely to appear. Dr. W. French Anderson and his colleagues at Washington, D.C.'s National Institutes of Health, the world's most prestigious health research facilities, undertook the first human gene–therapy experiment in 1990. The patient was a four-year-old girl with an enzyme deficiency disorder. A decade later, Dr. Anderson still sees much to be done. His prediction is that by 2025, "gene therapy will be revolutionizing medicine, in that most major diseases will have gene-therapy treatments." This revolution will not begin with the bang of the French one; there will be no storming of the Bastille. Instead, gene therapies will emerge one at a time over the next two or three decades. Their impact will be profound, however, probably altering permanently the treatment of one major class of disease after another.

Patients have their hopes raised, often prematurely, by headlines about genetic-sequencing successes. The emergence of tests will be rapid. Sadly, treatments will take years after initial discoveries to be available to patients. This gap between discovery and practical application causes frustration for patients and their families. But despite the tension between hopes and realities, genetic testing and gene therapy are a good bet to radically reshape the real treatment options in the twenty-first century. The cost of and demand for gene therapy, however, is likely to place still more strain on health financing.

Conclusion

Sir Thomas More: *Would you cut down all the laws of England*
to go after the devil?

William Roper: *Yes, I would. . . .*

More: *And if you cut them down . . . do you really*
think you could stand upright in the winds
that would blow then?

— ROBERT BOLT, *A MAN FOR ALL SEASONS*,
ACT III (1961)

How will health care fare in these turbulent times? Some days the winds feel more like a howling gale of change. They are reshaping our most important and long-standing forms of health care. The stand-alone hospital, the solo-practice physician, and the hospital-based nurse are formidable opponents, and the question as to whether these and other elements of the entrenched provider system can continue to stand upright is an open one. The result of this struggle, whatever it is, will be the emergent health system of the twenty-first century. Only the initial outlines of that new beast are yet evident; much more is to be revealed.

As we enter a new century, our four winds will continue to reshape the ways health services are conceived, defined, and delivered. Powerful ideas, such as determinants of health, are shifting and broadening the scope of health organizations. New information technologies are driving the measurement and management of outcomes. Greater public expectations relating to quality, speed, and appropriateness pose a formidable force for reform. Meanwhile, amidst the economic prosperity of the late 1990s, finances remain tight for health services. Pressures continue to find cost efficiencies.

The relative velocity of these four winds may alter. Finance may become a less powerful force than technology. We may face a decade with fewer new ideas in health policy and more emphasis on successful implementation of existing ideas. Public expectations, boosted by the aging baby boomers and fueled by Internet information sources, are likely to continue to rise.

The three-way tug of war among those who pay for health services, those who provide them, and those who receive them will not abate. In the United States, HMOs are not likely to be abolished — but they are likely to face tougher regulations. In the United Kingdom, Prime Minister Tony Blair will moderate, but not reverse, the internal-market reforms to the National Health Service. Canada's provinces will make changes to their regional health authorities, but they will continue to be the prevailing model of health-care funding and delivery.

Throughout the industrialized world, the return to strong economic growth will encourage reinvestment in health services. This will lead to more debate about where in the system money should be spent, and what appropriate targets are. The first decade of the twenty-first century will see these debates become more detailed and more focused on operational matters.

Technological progress offers us the prospect of great advances in the treatment and prevention of illness. Our true challenge is to put this river of information to work with wisdom and compassion. If we can meet it, we can alleviate much suffering and make billions of lives healthier.

Many involved in health services fear the financial consequences of expanding technology. Will health-service financing crumble under the sustained burden of a rapidly growing, frail, elderly population? Will aging boomers crush the financial stability of health care with their aggressive demands for speed and quality? Certainly the challenges posed by aging populations in North America and Europe will be formidable.

The old, familiar forms of health-care delivery — the hospital and the physicians' office — are transforming. In their place we have the health Web site on the Internet, the local health clinic, and the large, integrated health system. This transformation of delivery organizations will ultimately improve care services.

Many of those who work in health policy and management lament the pressures brought to bear on them daily by the emotive headlines in our newspapers. Rarely is "health care" included in a front-page headline without the word "crisis" nearby. Each case of delay or calamity for a patient is, after all, news. Newspapers, TV, and radio stations depend on the interest of their audiences — that is, us. Every failure of the health system is of interest, just as every passenger airplane or train that crashes is of interest.

Hysterical headlines do not make good health policy, but they are inevitable. Just as sure a thing are the stories touting miracle cures for cancer or diabetes, often based on very early research results. These are twin perils. An individual problem is transformed through the alchemy of the front page into a system-wide crisis; promising studies involving mice become instant cures for disease according to the evening television news. One clear lesson from this phenomenon is that those leading health organizations, whether they are in elected office or in management, need to be better and more frequent communicators. Only with diligent, patient explanation will an increasingly anxious public become informed and confident.

The twenty-first century will witness the coming of twin revolutions in health and health care, driven by the silicon chip and gene therapy. My imagination can sketch only the early outlines of the resulting transformation. The shift of health services from the hospital setting to the clinic and the home has only begun. Diagnostic and monitoring devices, ever smaller, cheaper, and more accurate, will support an extraordinary level of self-care by individuals. The unbundling of information from providers, already a key driver of Internet health sites, will go even further.

Speed will alter care services. General Electric's new "Light Speed" imaging scanner requires only thirty seconds to produce a patient's image, whereas existing MRIs need twenty minutes. This acceleration in the pace of diagnosis and treatment will alter health services. Enhanced speed is the answer to waiting lists and impatient patients; new, faster technologies coupled with a reordered health system will provide a counterbalance to an aging population with growing health-care needs.

Specific procedures, such as laser eye surgery, are moving out of the hospital setting. Clinics focused on specific procedures will be a growth sector. Eye clinics, foot clinics, back clinics, men's health and women's health centres are all on the horizon. As the twin technological revolutions create new, less-intensive procedures, these clinics will take up more of the burden of care, improving as they compete on the basis of speed, quality, and price.

What Does the Future Hold for Providers?

Rapid change in technologies in health will continue to challenge doctors and nurses. New, faster computers tracking health information and outcomes will provide benchmarks and comparisons. New drugs will require careful management. Overall, the potential for benefits to patients will steadily increase. The difficulties associated with actually bringing these benefits to patients are likely to increase as well, however.

Doctors, nurses, and others will need to become continual learners to keep pace. Old ways of delivering care will change.

Consider for a moment the traditional patient-doctor office visit. Historically a relatively low-tech encounter, it involved routine testing of blood pressure and often not much else. A few notes in the patient's record. Perhaps a prescription for a persistent rash or a stubborn cough. Contrast this with the future, when electronic patient records will be the norm. Non-invasive testing of breath, saliva, and sweat will allow a much more detailed picture of the patient's state of health. As well, the doctor-nurse team will be under pressure to enroll patients in a variety of organized disease-management programs. Preventive interventions such as smoking cessation and weight loss will be normal procedures as well.

The expectations placed on doctors are likely to race ahead of the financial incentives needed to fulfill them. More robust doctor-patient interaction at the primary-care level requires a complete overhaul of the solo-physician practice system with its low-tech offices, and an expansion of the nursing role — in short, more change.

Health-care providers are in for a turbulent decade — another one — as health-care delivery systems are reshaped around them. Morale will be hard to keep up. The pressure will cause a minority of providers to embrace extreme reform proposals. A better course of action, however, will be to advocate measures that improve the lot of patients, wherever possible.

What Does the Future Hold for Patients?

The good news for patients is that there will be more care options. Both where care can be obtained and what range of treatment options is available are expanding. The Internet-based health-information boom is more good news for patients. But the news is not all good. Increased options mean more complex systems and more difficult choices. The benefits of being well informed increase with the complexity of choices. The turmoil of this period of restructuring has disrupted the old relationships between patient and health services. In this period of accelerated change, it is not surprising that public confidence in the system has been undermined. The old level of trust in the system is unlikely to be completely restored, but as its performance improves, some confidence will be regained.

Early evidence suggests that new health-services organizations will have two primary mandates. First, they will continue in the time-honoured task of providing health services to the ill and injured. Aging populations will accelerate demand for these services. But as a second, no less important mission, these new, larger health organizations will focus on the health of the population. It is this mandate that distinguishes the integrated or regional health organization from the hospital, and represents a profound change in the health world. To date, there is more evidence of success than failure in this shift.

You will recognize these new organizations in your city or neighbourhood. They have names like University Health Network, Regional Health Authority, or Integrated Health System. What differentiates them from the hospitals they are replacing is that to them, you are not just a potential patient but a "preventable patient." Efforts will be expended to keep you in better health, even if you never see the inside of a hospital in your life. From smoking-cessation classes to disease-management programs for asthma, diabetes, or arthritis patients, various forms of support will spring up to help us all live healthier lives.

This trend is not one of altruism. Those in today's health system know that the cost of your health care will decrease if you live a healthier life. As well, your health payer, whether employer or government, has embraced the concept of broader determinants of health and will make you aware of this fact in a variety of ways. More efforts individually tailored to meet your health needs will be evident; enhanced electronic health records will replace paper files; you will know much more about your body, including its genetic strengths and weaknesses. Innovations devoted to increasing your health and well-being — and also to your appearance — will abound, from hair-growth medications to teeth whiteners to new-age orthotics for your feet.

What Kind of System Will the Winds Bring?

The problem of providing high-quality health services to any population will not be completely solved. Managing health-care services is truly life in a puzzle factory; at least it is never dull work. The challenges posed by a demanding citizenry, evolving technology, and the traditional resistance of health-care organizations to change are serious. Those who make health-care policy are in for another decade of a difficult balancing act. This tension is properly perceived as the management of changing, expanding public expectations in a context of increasing possibilities. The answer is not unlimited funding or unpalatable rationing. It is a more informed patient, and a realistic attitude about what can possibly be provided to all. The health needs of our populations can be met, but perhaps not all the health-care demands. Discerning the difference between them will be, as it has always been, more of an art than a science.

Good health remains a goal for each individual, family, community, and nation. The tools, technologies, and insights at our disposal to achieve this goal are more powerful then they have been at any previous time in the lengthy history of our species. How well will we use this newfound power? Will we put new vaccines to work in the least developed nations? Are we able to take a global view? Led by international agencies such as the World Health Organization, the United Nations, and its Population Council, I believe the appropriate answer is yes. Perhaps the biggest impact of the Internet and television will be to create Marshall McLuhan's "global village."

Currently, our globe may be a village, but it is one with an unacceptable degree of difference between the health of our wealthiest and that of our poorest citizens. We know how to reduce these disparities. In his book *Walter Benjamin at the Dairy Queen: Reflections at Sixty and Beyond* American novelist Larry McMurtry wrote:

> The sin that television journalism singly must answer for is that of bringing the unredeemed pain of the whole planet into our daily

lives. A village is buried by a mudslide in Peru. We see the small, hopeless people probing the mud which has just buried their homes and killed their children.

Perhaps within this sin there is the blessing that will lead us to a more determined international effort to improve the health of all peoples in all nations. There *should* be such an effort. If television hastens its coming, it can be forgiven many other sins.

The four winds of health-care change, properly harnessed, can move health systems in the developed nations forward, toward a broader purpose and more effective operations. As forces of change, the winds in and of themselves are neither virtuous nor destructive. It is the skill of the sailor that determines the outcome of wind on sails. So, too, will it be the navigational skills of all of us in health policy, health management, and health provision that determine where our health systems ultimately end up.

I remain an optimist about the future of health services. Despite the trauma that always accompanies changes, I believe we are all learning to steer our craft into the wind. We are also designing systems that are lighter, more flexible, and closer to the populations they serve. We have the potential to create faster services, with higher and more measurable quality. I believe our health systems will bend and be reshaped, but ultimately remain upright in the winds that are blowing.

Glossary of Terms

acute care — Care for those with acute, or very serious, health conditions.

Canadian Institute for Health Information (CIHI) — A national non-profit organization that is working to develop a set of indicators to measure and track the health of Canadians.

carcinogen — An agent, such as a chemical or radiation, that causes cancer.

clinical epidemiology — The study of the outcomes resulting from clinical interventions, or, more often, the study of the patterns of those outcomes.

Cochrane Collaboration — An international group that compiles systematic, up-to-date reviews of relevant, randomized clinical trials of health care.

Crown health enterprises — New Zealand organizations; the cornerstone of its approach to more integrated delivery of health services.

DNA — Deoxyribonucleic acid; the nucleotide polymer that carries
genetic information.

demand management — The effort to reduce health-care costs by
reducing the need and demand for medical service.

disability-adjusted life year — An estimate of an individual's life span
based on health factors.

disease-state management — An approach that coordinates health-care
resources for patients for the duration of their diseases.

evidence-based medicine — An approach that focuses on measuring
outcomes and assessing the value of medical interventions
scientifically.

gene — A unit of heredity, a region of DNA that controls a discreet
hereditary characteristic; a gene is the "recipe" that controls
production of a specific protein, and includes regulatory signals.

genetic code — The language — universal to all life on Earth — in
which genetic instructions are written to direct protein production.
Each triplet of four nucleotides codes for one of 20 amino acids, or
a stop signal.

genetics — The scientific study of how traits are transmitted from
parents to offspring.

genome — The totality of genetic information belonging to an organism, its set of genes. The human genome is defined within 24
chromosomes — the 22 autosomes plus the two sex chromosomes.

health maintenance organization (HMO) — A medical network management company that operates multi-specialty medical clinics
and independent practice associations, and provides health-care
decision-support services to consumers.

horizontal integration — The combining of similar organizations; for
example, the merger of two hospitals.

integrated health network — A network of acute-care hospitals.

integrated health systems — An extensive integration of health services.

Magnetic Resonance Imagery (MRI) — Technology that uses a spectrometer to produce electronic images of the inside of the human body.

managed care — Health care that is provided with an emphasis on efficiency, and thus reduced costs.

managed competition — An approach based on the notion that competition drives efficiency in the health-care system.

meta-analysis — A statistical method of synthesizing research results.

National Health Service — The national organization delivering health care in Great Britain; a nationwide, organized health system that strives to apply uniform standards of service and coverage.

pharmaceutical-benefits management — The organized management of drug benefits; generally undertaken by third-party firms.

population health — The health of a population as a whole.

primary care — The provision of integrated, accessible health-care services by clinicians who are accountable for addressing a large majority of personal health-care needs, developing a sustained partnership with patients, and practising in the context of family and community.

regionalization — The defining of geographical regions and creation of health-care services organizations based upon those boundaries.

sequence — The particular order of nucleotides in DNA or of amino acids in a protein. The sequence is an identifying "signature."

silicon chip — A computer chip that provides the technology to obtain, store, and manage information.

telehealth — The use of communications and information technology to deliver health services, products, and education through networks and databases.

vertical integration — The combining of different organizations; for example, a doctor's clinic and a hospital.

World Bank — An international bank that administers economic aid among member nations of the United Nations.

World Health Organization (WHO) — A United Nations agency that promotes health and controls communicable diseases.

Select Bibliography

Boston Consulting Group. *The Promise of Disease Management.* Chicago: Boston Consulting Group, 1995.

Brown, S., and D. Grimes. *Nurse Practitioners and Certified Nurse-Midwives: A Meta-analysis of Studies in Primary Care Roles.* Washington, D.C.: American Nurses Publishing, 1993.

Canadian College of Health Service Executives (CCHSE). *Health Reform Update, 1997/98.* Ottawa: CCHSE, undated: 1–12.

Central Sydney Area Health Service. *Annual Report, 1994/95.* Sydney, Australia: Central Sydney Area Health Service, 1995.

Cochrane A.L. *Effectiveness and Efficiency: Random Reflections on Health Services.* London, UK: Nuffield Provincial Hospitals Trust, 1972. (Reprinted in 1989 in association with *The British Medical Journal.*)

——. "1931–1971: A Critical Review, with Particular Reference to the Medical Profession." In *Medicines for the Year 2000.* London, UK:

Office of Health Economics, 1979, 1–11.

Crosby, F., M.R. Ventura, and M.J. Feldman. "Future Research Recommendations for Establishing Nurse Practitioner Effectiveness." *Nurse Practitioner* 12(1) 1987: 75–79.

Decter, Michael. *Healing Medicare: Managing Health System Change the Canadian Way*. Toronto: McGilligan Books, 1994.

Donelan, Karen, et al. "The Cost of Health System Change: Public Discontent in Five Nations." Data Watch. *Health Affairs* May/June 1999: 206–16.

Durham, G. "Public Health and Disease Prevention — Moving Forward in New Zealand and Australia: Public Health Framework in New Zealand." *Health Care Review — Online* 3(7).
http://www.enigma.co.nz/hcro-articles/9907/vol3no7-001.htm

Evans, R.G., M. Barer, and T. Marmor (eds.). *Why Are Some People Healthy and Others Not?: The Determinants of Health of Populations*. New York: Aldine de Gruyter, 1994.

Fitzmartin, Ronald D. "The Driving Forces for Global Technological and Process Change." *Drug Information Journal* 1998 32: 859–60.

Foot, David, and Daniel Stoffman. *Boom, Bust, and Echo 2000: Profiting from the Demographic Shift in the New Millennium*. Toronto: Macfarlane, Walter and Ross, 1998.

Forget, Monique Jerome, and Claude E. Forget. *Who Is the Master?: A Blueprint for Canadian Health Care Reform*. Montreal, Quebec: Institute for Research on Public Policy, 1998.

Fry, James C., Everett Coop, Carson Beadle, et al. "Reducing Health-Care Costs by Reducing the Need and Demand for Medical Services." *New England Journal of Medicine* 329(5) (29 July 1993): 321–25.

Glouberman, Sholom, et al. "A New Perspective on Health Policy." Presentation to the Policy Research Network, June 28, 1999, Ottawa.

Griffiths, Jenny. "Whose Health Service Is it Anyway?: An 'up over' Experience of Health Service Evolution." Paper presented to the Australian College of Health Service Executives and RACMA Congress, August 28–30, 1996, Darwin, Australia.

Hamilton, Nancy, and Tariq Bhatti. *Population Health Promotion: An*

Integrated Model of Population Health and Health Promotion. Ottawa: Health Canada, Health Promotion Development Division, 1996.

Hastings, Fiona (ed.). *Beyond Provider Dominance.* London, U.K.: King's Fund, 1994.

Health and Welfare Canada. *A New Perspective on the Health of Canadians.* Ottawa, Ontario: Health and Welfare Canada, 1974.

———. *Achieving Health for All: A Framework for Health Promotion.* Ottawa, Ontario: Health and Welfare Canada, 1986.

Health Canada, Federal, Provincial, and Territorial Advisory Committee on Population Health. *Strategies for Population Health.* Ottawa, Ontario: Health Canada, 1999.

———. *Toward a Healthy Future.* Ottawa, Ontario: Health Canada, 1998.

Health Canada, Office of Health and the Information Highway Policy and Consultation Branch. *Tele-Homecare: An Overview Background Paper for Discussion.* Ottawa, Ontario: Health Canada, 1999.

Health Care International. *Healthcare Industry, 3rd Quarter 1999.* London, U.K.: The Economist Intelligence Unit, 1999.

"The Health Field Concept Then and Now: Snapshots of Canada." *Towards a New Perspective on Health Policy.* Working Paper #1. Ottawa, Ontario: Canadian Research Network, 1999.

Hertzlinger, Regina, *Market Driven Health Care.* Reading, Massachusetts: Addison Wesley, 1996.

Hirji, Zenita, and Andrew Holt. "Hospitals in the U.K. Health System." *Hospital Quarterly* Fall 1997.

Knieps, Franz. "The Present Situation of Non-Primary Care, Especially Hospital Care, in Germany: Remarks from a Fund's Point of View." Paper given at Four-Country Conference in Bonn, Germany, AOK-Bundesverband, 1997.

Knowles, David. "Policy Developments: British Healthcare Reform Through Internal Markets and Beyond." Paper presented to the OHA Convention, Toronto, November 4, 1997.

Labonte, R. "Population Health and Health Promotion: What Do They Have to Say to Each Other?" *Canadian Journal of Public Health* 86(3) 1995: 165–68.

_____. "Health Promotion: From Concepts to Strategies." *Healthcare Management Forum* 1988 (Autumn): 24–30.

Lalonde, Marc. *A New Perspective on the Health of Canadians: A Working Document.* (The Lalonde Report.) Ottawa, Ontario: Health and Welfare Canada, 1974.

Leatt, Peggy, George H. Pink, and C. David Naylor. "Integrated Delivery Systems: Has Their Time Come in Canada?" *Canadian Medical Association Journal* 1996 (March 15).

Maclean's. The Health Report. June 15, 1998.

_____. *The Health Report.* October 25, 1999.

Maxwell, Dr. Robert J. "Beyond Restructuring: The Limit of Simple Fixes." Paper presented to the OHA Convention, Toronto, November 4, 1997.

Merck-Frosst Canada and Coalition of Voluntary Organizations. *Canadian Health Care Survey.* Toronto: Merck-Frosst Canada, 1998.

Metropolitan Toronto District Health Council (MTDHC). *Planning, Funding, and Managing Metropolitan Toronto's Health System: Options for the Future.* Action Plan 7. Toronto: MTDHC, 1995.

_____. *Toward a Healthier Tomorrow: Strategies for Promoting Health in Metro Toronto.* Report of the MTDHC Health Promotion and Strategic Policy Committee. Toronto: MTDHC, 1996.

Molloy, Dr. William. *Vital Choices: Life, Death, and the Health-Care Crises.* Toronto: Penguin Books, 1994.

Noseworthy, T.W. "Canada Deserves a National Health System." *Health-Care Management Forum* 10(1): 39–46.

Ontario Health Services Restructuring Commission. *A Vision of Ontario's Health Services System.* Report. Toronto: Health Services Restructuring Commission, January 1997.

Ontario Nurses' Association. *Dialogue on Health Reform*, Ontario Nurses' Association, Toronto (Summer 1996).

Owen, John Wyn. *Health Care Reforms in New South Wales.* Paper presented to 1996 Australian College of Health Service Executives and RACMA Congress, August 28–30, 1996, Darwin, Australia.

Pointer, Dennis D., Jeffrey A. Alexander, and Howard S. Zuckerman. "Loosening the Gordian Knot of Governance in Integrated Health Care Delivery Systems." *Frontiers of Health Services Manager* 11:3.

Priest, Lisa. *Operating in the Dark*. Toronto: Doubleday, 1998.

Rovin, Sheldon, et al. *An Idealized Design of the U.S. Health-Care System*. Bryn Mawr, Pennsylvania: Interact, The Institute for Interactive Management, 1994.

Saskatoon Regional Health District (SRHD). *Annual Report, 1994/95*. Saskatoon, Saskatchewan: SRHD, 1995.

Shah, C.P. *Public Health and Preventive Medicine in Canada. Third edition*. Toronto: University of Toronto Press, 1994. See especially Chapter 1, "Concepts, Determinants, and Promotion of Health," pp. 3–26; Chapter 4, "Determinants of Health and Disease," pp. 79–99; and "Emerging Issues in Health Care Delivery," pp. 377–98.

Shortell, Stephen M., Robin R. Gillies, and David A. Anderson. "The New World of Managed Care: Creating Organized Delivery Systems." *Health Affairs*, Winter 1994.

Singer, Dr. Peter. *Living Will*. Toronto: Centre for Bioethics, University of Toronto 1994. Includes forms.

Statistics Canada. *Health Reports* 2(2) (Autumn 1999).

Stoelwinder, J. "Against the Odds? Integrating Care in a Multi-Payer Health System. A Case Study." Paper presented to the King's Fund International Seminar, Toronto, 1997.

Tapscott, Don. *The Digital Economy: Promise and Peril in the Age of Networked Intelligence*. New York: McGraw Hill, 1996. Particularly pp. 125–31 on the subject of digital health.

United Kingdom, Department of Health. *A Guide to the National Health Service*. London, U.K.: NHS Executive Communications Unit, 1996.

United Kingdom, Secretary of State for Health. *Health of the Nation*. London, U.K.: Queen's Printer, 1992.

United Nations Development Program. *Human Development Report 1998*. New York: Oxford University Press, 1998.

Wit Capital. *Wit's Wisdom on eHealth*. Particularly Issue #4 (May 26,

1999) and Issue #6 (October 18, 1999). www.witcapital.com

World Bank. *World Development Report 1993: Investing in Health.* Washington, D.C.: World Bank, 1993.

World Health Organization, Health and Welfare Canada, and Canadian Public Health Association (CPHA). *Ottawa Charter for Health Promotion.* Ottawa, Ontario: CPHA, 1986.

Index